Sexual and
Reproductive Health
at a Glance

This title is also available as an e-book.
For more details, please see
www.wiley.com/buy/9781118460726
or scan this QR code:

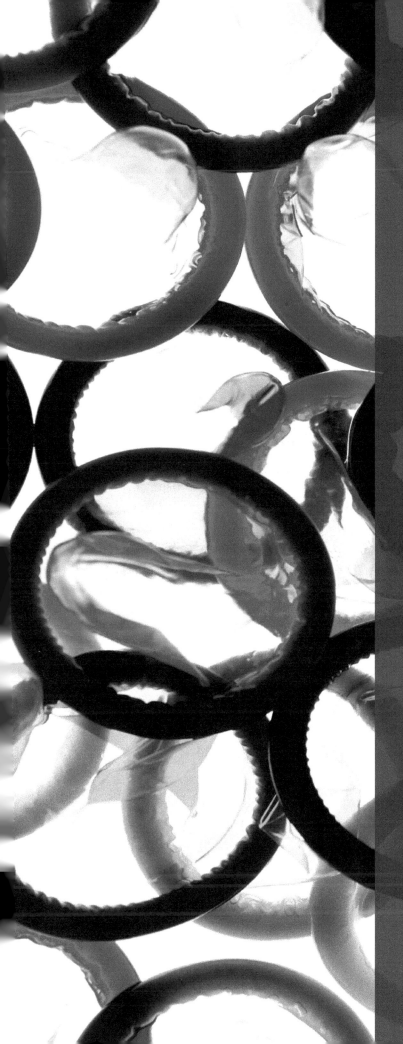

Sexual and Reproductive Health
at a Glance

Catriona Melville

MSc FRCOG MFSRH DipGUM

Consultant in Sexual and Reproductive Health
NHS Ayrshire and Arran

The Gatehouse, Ayrshire Central Hospital
Scotland, United Kingdom

WILEY Blackwell

This edition first published 2015 © 2015 John Wiley & Sons Ltd

Registered Office
John Wiley & Sons Ltd, The Atrium, Southern Gate, Chichester, West Sussex, PO19 8SQ, UK

Editorial Offices
9600 Garsington Road, Oxford, OX4 2DQ, UK
350 Main Street, Malden, MA 02148-5020, USA
111 River Street, Hoboken, NJ 07030-5774, USA
The Atrium, Southern Gate, Chichester, West Sussex, PO19 8SQ, UK

For details of our global editorial offices, for customer services and for information about how to apply for permission to reuse the copyright material in this book please see our website at www.wiley.com/wiley-blackwell.

Library of Congress Cataloging-in-Publication Data
Melville, Catriona, author.
  Sexual and reproductive health at a glance / Catriona Melville.
    p. ; cm.
  Includes bibliographical references and index.
  ISBN 978-1-118-46072-6 (pbk.)
  I. Title.
  [DNLM: 1. Reproductive Health. 2. Contraception. 3. Genital Diseases, Female. 4. Sexual Dysfunction, Physiological. 5. Sexually Transmitted Diseases. WQ 200.1]
  RA788
  613.9—dc23
                    2014032707

A catalogue record for this book is available from the British Library.

Cover image: iStock © pederk

Set in 9.5/11.5pt Minion Pro by SPi Global, Chennai, India

Printed and bound by CPI Group (UK) Ltd, Croydon, CR0 4YY

C9781118460726_240924

Contents

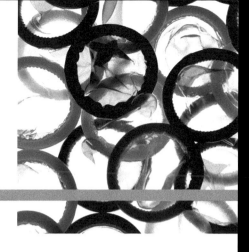

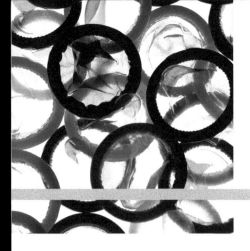

Acknowledgements

Thanks to Mark Mason, Senior Specialist Biomedical Scientist, Sandyford, NHS Greater Glasgow & Clyde, Glasgow, UK, for the images reproduced from Sandyford.

I would like to extend my gratitude to family, friends and colleagues on both sides of the globe who offered feedback or acted as a sounding board while I was undertaking this project.

I would also like to thank my husband Rory and my children Dougray and Angus for their unconditional and immeasurable support, patience and encouragement which I found invaluable during the writing of this text book.

Catriona Melville

Abbreviations

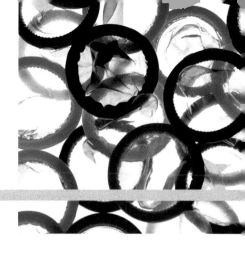

AEDs	antiepileptic drugs	EC	emergency contraception
AIDs	acquired immunodeficiency syndrome	ECG	electrocardiogram
AIN	anal intraepithelial neoplasia	ED	erectile dysfunction
ALF	acute liver failure	EE	ethinylestradiol
ART	antiretroviral therapy	EIs	entry inhibitors
ALO	actinomyces-like organisms	ENG	etonogestrel
AUB	abnormal uterine bleeding	EP	ectopic pregnancy
BASHH	British Association for Sexual Health and HIV	EPR	electronic patient record
		ESR	erythrocyte sedimentation rate
BBT	basal body temperature	EVA	electric vacuum aspiration
BBV	blood-borne viruses	FAM	fertility awareness method
BFPR	biological false positive reaction	FBC	full blood count
BHIVA	British HIV Association	FIGO	International Federation of Gynecology and Obstetrics
BMD	bone mineral density		
BMI	body mass index	FME	forensic medical examination
BNF	British National Formulary	FPU	Family Protection Unit
BPAS	British Pregnancy Advisory Service	FSH	follicular stimulating hormone
BTB	breakthrough bleeding	FSRH	Faculty of Sexual and Productive Healthcare
BV	bacterial vaginosis	FVU	first void urine
CBT	cognitive behavioural therapy	GnRH	gonadotrophin-releasing hormone
CD	Crohn's disease	GMC	General Medical Council
CEU	Clinical Effectiveness Unit	GUD	genital ulcer disease
CHCs	combined hormonal contraceptives	GUM	Genitourinary Medicine
CIN	cervical intra-epithelial neoplasia	GBV	gender based violence
CMO	Chief Medical Officer	HAART	highly active antiretroviral therapy
COC	combined oral contraceptive	HAV	hepatitis A virus
CPP	chronic pelvic pain	HBV	hepatitis B virus
CRP	C-reactive protein	HCP	healthcare professional
CSF	cerebrospinal fluid	HCV	hepatitis C virus
CSRH	Community Sexual and Reproductive Health	HERS	Heart and Estrogen/Progestin Replacement Study
CT	computerized tomography		
CTP	combined transdermal patch	HCG	human chorionic gonadotrophin
Cu-IUD	copper intrauterine device	HIV	human immunodeficiency virus
CVD	cardiovascular disease	HIV PEPSE	HIV post-exposure prophylaxis after sexual exposure
CVR	combined vaginal ring		
CXR	chest X-ray	HMB	heavy menstrual bleeding
D&E	dilatation and evacuation	HPS	Health Protection Scotland
DH	Department of Health	HPV	human papilloma virus
DGI	disseminated gonococcal infection	HRT	hormone replacement therapy
DMPA	depot medroxyprogesterone acetate	HSV	herpes simplex virus
DNG	dienogest	HVS	high vaginal swab
DRSP	Daily Record of Severity of Problems	IBD	inflammatory bowel disease
DUB	dysfunctional uterine bleeding	IIs	integrase inhibitors
E2V	estradiol valerate	IM	intramuscular
EAGA	Expert Advisory Group on AIDS	IMB	intermenstrual bleeding

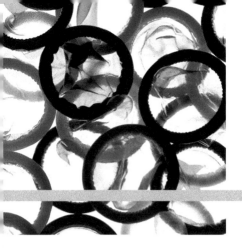

About the companion website

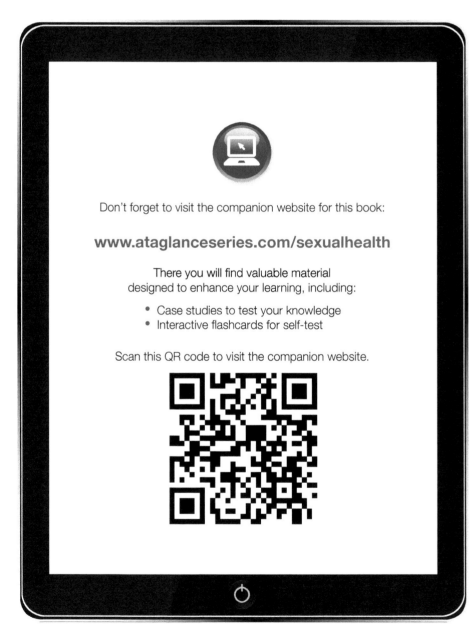

Don't forget to visit the companion website for this book:

www.ataglanceseries.com/sexualhealth

There you will find valuable material
designed to enhance your learning, including:

- Case studies to test your knowledge
- Interactive flashcards for self-test

Scan this QR code to visit the companion website.

Principles of sexual and reproductive health

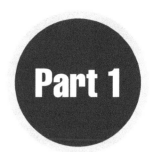

Part 1

Chapter

 Don't forget to visit the companion website at www.ataglanceseries.com/sexualhealth where you can test yourself on these topics.

Table 1.1   UKMEC categories

UKMEC 1	A condition for which there is no restriction for the use of the method
UKMEC 2	A condition where the advantages of using the method generally outweigh the risks
UKMEC 3	A condition where the risks of using the method usually outweigh the advantages (see text for further explanation)
UKMEC 4	A condition which represents an unacceptable health risk if the method is used

Table 1.2   LARC methods

Contraceptive method	Duration of action for contraception	Pregnancy rate
Cu-IUD	5 – 10 years	< 20 in 1000 over 5 years*
LNG-IUS	5 years	< 10 in 1000 over 5 years
Progestogen-only implant e.g. Nexplanon	3 years	< 4 in 1000 over 2 years
Progestogen-only injection e.g. DMPA	12 weeks for IM-DMPA, 13 weeks for SC-DMPA (8 weeks for NET-EN)	< 1 in 1000 over 3 years

* for devices containing 380 mm² copper

Figure 1.2   Hypothalamic-pituitary-ovarian axis

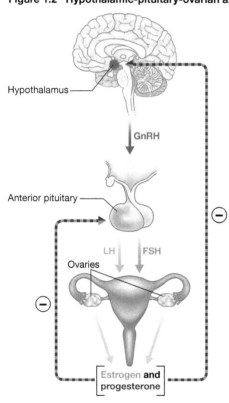

Figure 1.3   Female reproductive cycle

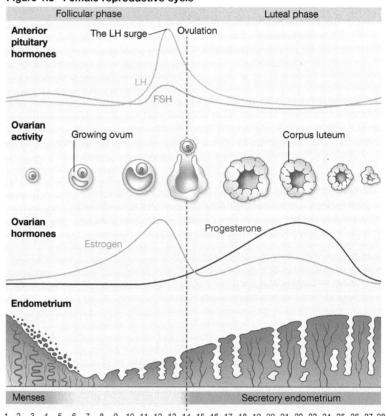

UKMEC

The UK Medical Eligibility Criteria (UKMEC) for Contraceptive Use were adapted from the World Health Organization Medical Eligibility Criteria (WHOMEC) to provide evidence-based guidance for the safe use of contraceptives in the presence of specific characteristics or medical conditions. UKMEC has four categories. The definitions are given in Table 1.1.

In practical terms, a UKMEC category of 1 or 2 would allow safe use of the contraceptive method; conditions given a category 3 would only allow the method to be used if other methods are unacceptable or unavailable and on the advice of a specialist contraceptive provider, and category 4 indicates that the method is contraindicated with this condition.

Additionally, some methods are awarded different categories to distinguish between initiation of the method (I) and continuation of the method (C). For example, if a client requests insertion of a copper intrauterine device (Cu-IUD) (initiation) but has untreated chlamydia infection, this would be awarded a UKMEC category 4 (until the condition has been treated); if however a client is diagnosed with chlamydia infection and has a Cu-IUD already in situ then continuation of this method is a UKMEC 2.

UKMEC also provides categories for fertility based awareness methods and for male and female sterilization (see individual chapters for details).

Long-acting reversible methods (LARC) (Table 1.2)

- LARC methods are contraceptive methods which are administered less than once per cycle or month
- These methods do not depend on daily adherence and therefore offer higher efficacy than methods such as the combined oral contraceptive pill (COC) or progestogen-only pill (POP)
- Increasing the uptake of LARC can reduce the number of unintended pregnancies
- Despite the initial higher outlay (in terms of cost of method and staff time), the LARC methods are more cost-effective even at 1 year than the COC
- The very-long-acting methods (vLARC), namely the intrauterine methods and the progestogen only implant are more cost-effective than the progestogen-only injectable
- Service providers should offer women a choice of contraceptive methods including LARC

Partner notification

Partner notification (PN) is an essential component of care, which should be provided by all services managing sexually transmitted infections (STIs). PN (also called contact tracing) is a mechanism whereby the sexual contacts (past and/or present) of a person with a diagnosed STI (the index case) are informed in order that they can access appropriate advice, testing and treatment. Each STI has a look-back interval in which infection of sexual contacts may have occurred. The aims of PN are:

- to prevent reinfection of the index case
- to prevent the sequelae of undiagnosed infection in sexual contacts
- to prevent the onward transmission of STIs in the community (a Public Health issue)

Partners can be informed by the patient themselves (index referral) or by health professionals (provider referral). Newer strategies aimed at improving PN rates are being studied, e.g. using patient-delivered testing kits or patient-delivered partner therapy (PDPT). In the UK PN is voluntary; however, in other countries such as Norway and Sweden it is compulsory (a legal requirement).

Staff in SRH services

SRH services are consultant led, but the role of nurses has evolved, and experienced nurse practitioners staff many clinics independently or alongside medical colleagues. Additionally, healthcare assistants often provide sexual health screening to 'low risk', asymptomatic patients.

Sexual health advisors have an important role within an SRH service. They provide information, advice and counselling to patients diagnosed with an STI. They facilitate PN and support patients in managing their condition. They provide sexual health education and health promotion and a range of counselling interventions. In some services, this role will be undertaken by a practitioner with sexual health advising competencies.

Notifiable diseases

The Health Protection (Notification) Regulations 2010 (Department of Health, England) outline the responsibilities to notify the proper officer of a local authority of individual cases of specified infectious diseases. In Northern Ireland, England and Wales, acute hepatitis A, B and C are notifiable diseases. In Scotland, under the Public Health etc. (Scotland) Act 2008, hepatitis is not notifiable by clinicians; however, hepatitis A, B and C are notifiable organisms and diagnostic laboratories must report identification of these viruses to Health Protection Scotland (HPS).

'Off-label' prescribing

Practical prescribing of contraceptives and other drugs in SRH, may be at odds with the product licence. The GMC offers guidance for such 'off-label' prescribing in 'Good Practice in Prescribing Medicines' (2008). 'Off-label' use in these situations is sanctioned as long as there is sufficient evidence base for such use. Furthermore, if such use is deemed 'common practice' then documentation regarding non-licensed use, may not be required on every occasion. Evidence based guidance from National Institute for Health and Care Excellence (NICE) and the FSRH are examples of accepted 'common practice'.

The female reproductive cycle (Figures 1.2, 1.3)

- The female reproductive (menstrual) cycle is controlled by the anterior pituitary hormones luteinizing hormone (LH) and follicular stimulating hormone (FSH), which are regulated via the hypothalamic secretion of gonadotrophin-releasing hormone (GnRH)
- LH and FSH stimulate the release of the ovarian hormones estrogen and progesterone
- The average reproductive cycle length is 28 days but it can vary from 21 to 35 days
- Day 1 is the first day of menstruation
- The follicular phase is from day 1of the cycle until ovulation and is of variable length
- The luteal phase is from ovulation until the next menses and its duration is fairly constant at 14 days ±2 days. To calculate the approximate day of ovulation, 14 days should be subtracted from the total cycle length

Box 1.5   Risk factors for STIs

- Non-use of barrier method
- Multiple partners (≥ 2 partners in last year) or recent change in partner
- Age < 25 years
- Sexuality: men who have sex with men (MSM)
- Previous STI

Box 1.6   Assessing pregnancy risk

- Date of LMP
- Was it a normal period?
- Date of last sexual intercourse
- Contraception used reliably for last sexual intercourse (SI)?
- Emergency contraception used?

Box 1.7   Reliably excluding pregnancy

You can be 'reasonably certain' that pregnancy is excluded if ≥ 1 of the following criteria are met (and there are no signs or symptoms of pregnancy):

- No SI has occurred since the last normal menstrual period
- There has been correct and consistent use of a reliable contraceptive method
- The woman is:
  within the first 7 days of the onset of a normal menstrual period
  or < 4 weeks postpartum (not breastfeeding)
  or < 7 days post-abortion or miscarriage
- Fully or nearly fully breastfeeding, amenorrhoeic and < 6 months postpartum

N.B. A pregnancy test can help exclude pregnancy but only if ≥ 3 weeks since last UPSI

Further reading: http://www.fsrh.org/pdfs/SelectedPracticeRecommendations2002.pdf

Figure 1.4   Female external genitalia

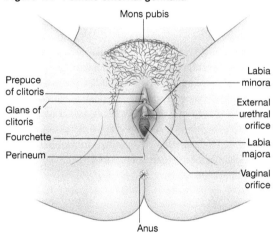

Mons pubis
Prepuce of clitoris
Glans of clitoris
Fourchette
Perineum
Labia minora
External urethral orifice
Labia majora
Vaginal orifice
Anus

Figure 1.5   Female reproductive system (lithotomy position)

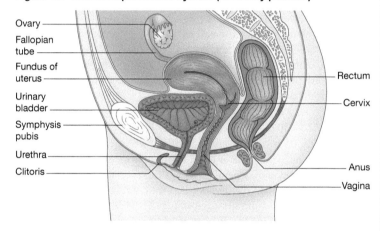

Ovary
Fallopian tube
Fundus of uterus
Urinary bladder
Symphysis pubis
Urethra
Clitoris
Rectum
Cervix
Anus
Vagina

Figure 1.6   Ventral image of penis

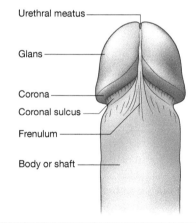

Urethral meatus
Glans
Corona
Coronal sulcus
Frenulum
Body or shaft

Figure 1.7   Male reproductive system

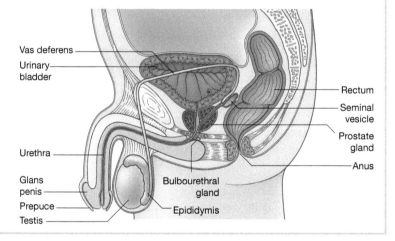

Vas deferens
Urinary bladder
Urethra
Glans penis
Prepuce
Testis
Bulbourethral gland
Epididymis
Rectum
Seminal vesicle
Prostate gland
Anus

History taking

Taking a concise history is a fundamental element of the SRH consultation. Many of the history taking skills overlap with those used in general consultations; however, there are specific aspects unique to SRH which must be included. As the sexual history necessitates enquiring about very personal issues, it is vital that the consultation takes place in a private environment with no interruptions. It is essential that the patient deems this a safe and confidential setting in which they can disclose intimate information.

Communication

Good communication skills and a non-judgemental approach are vital when working in an SRH setting. Clients can be extremely anxious or embarrassed. Explaining the rational for some of the questions you are asking may be helpful, e.g.

"Some of the questions I'm going to ask you today are quite personal but they are important to see how we can help you."

Open questions should be asked and non-verbal cues – particularly signs of distress – should be recognized.

Components of the SRH history

Reason for attendance

* *Presenting complaint and history of presenting complaint*: enquire specifically about symptoms, their onset and any treatments the patient may have already tried
* *Past medical, surgical and family history*
* *Drug history*: including allergies

Questions about the presenting complaint:

* Is there any urethral/vaginal discharge?
* Any genital lumps/bumps/ulcers/blisters?
* Any genital soreness
* Pain passing urine?
* Any abdominal pain or pain during sex?
* Abnormal vaginal bleeding?
* Is there any systemic upset?
* Is there a rash?

Reproductive history

* *Menstrual history*: LMP, menstrual problems (current or past), changes in bleeding pattern
* *Contraceptive history:* current contraceptive method (if any) and any problems with this? Barrier method used? Past contraceptive methods
* *Gynaecological and obstetric history*: number and outcome of previous pregnancies; cervical cytology screening and whether any previous colposcopy

Sexual history

* *Recent sexual history*: when did they last have sexual intercourse? What was the gender of that person? Was it a casual or regular partner? What kind of sexual contact did they have (oral, vagina, anal)? Did they use a barrier method of contraception and was it effective? How many partners have they had in the last 3 and 12 months, and how many of these were new partners?
* *Lifetime sexual history*: how many previous sexual partners have they had? Have their previous partners been male, female or both and how do they identify their sexuality. Have they had sex with someone from another country and if so which country? Have they ever had sex involving payment? Any history of STIs? Do they use barrier methods?
* *Blood-borne viruses (BBV)*: have they ever injected drugs or share needles or had sex with someone who has? Have they had blood transfusions at home or abroad or tattoos in an 'unsafe' environment? Have they ever been tested for HIV or hepatitis B or C (when and what was the result?). Have they been vaccinated for hepatitis B?

Social history

* *Smoking history*: important for contraception prescribing
* *Alcohol and recreational drug consumption*: identifies risk taking behaviours and gives an opportunity for brief interventions
* *Gender based violence (GBV)*: enquire about a history of domestic violence or bullying and any previous non-consensual sexual activity including childhood sexual abuse. Routine enquiry about current and historic GBV is mandatory in SH services in Scotland

Finally, it is useful to ask the patient what their concerns are. There may have been suspected infidelity in a relationship or they may be anxious about a (often inaccurate) self-diagnosis they have made. Enabling the client to express these concerns can be helpful. It is also useful to ask what treatments the patient has tried and what effect (if any) these have had.

Risk assessment (Boxes 1.5–1.7)

It is useful to gather your thoughts after taking the history and make a risk assessment from the information you have obtained. You should assess the risk of pregnancy, STIs and BBVs. Based on the history you should also be able to decide which tests should be offered to the patient (although sometimes your examination findings will alter this), and whether they will need to return for further tests in a set period of time (e.g. too early for accurate pregnancy testing, or within the window period for HIV testing). You should also be able to reliably exclude pregnancy.

Examination

Intimate examinations

A chaperone should be offered for all intimate examinations regardless of the gender of health care professional (HCP) or client. The presence of a chaperone and their identity should be documented in the client's case record. Permission for the examination should also be sought and documented.

Male and female reproductive anatomy (Figures 1.4–1.7)

Anatomical drawings are often used in history-taking pro formas to identify the site of lesions. Otherwise, any examination findings should be described as accurately as possible in relation to anatomical landmarks.

Box 1.8 Bimanual pelvic examination

- **Uterus:** direction (anteverted, retroverted or axial), size and mobility, tenderness
- **Adnexae:** normal or enlarged, any tenderness
- **Presence of pelvic masses**
- **Discomfort or pain:** does the examination elicit any tenderness, e.g. cervical motion pain?

Box 1.9 Routine STI screen (asymptomatic patients)

Tests for
Chlamydia
Syphilis
Gonorrhoea
HIV

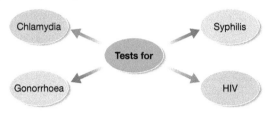

Figure 1.8 On-site microscopy

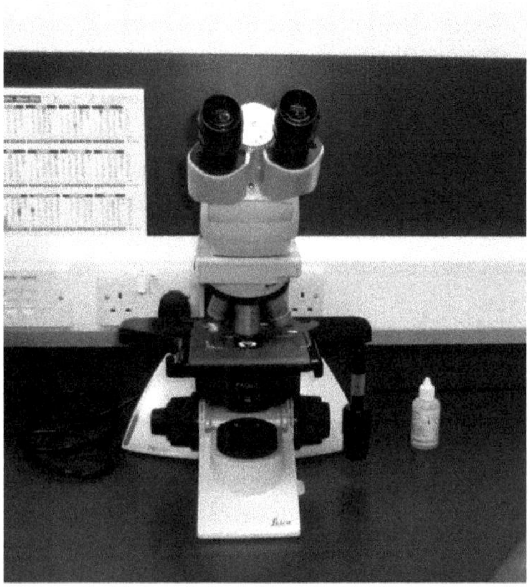

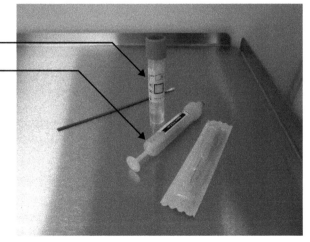

Figure 1.9 Self-taken vulvo-vaginal swab method

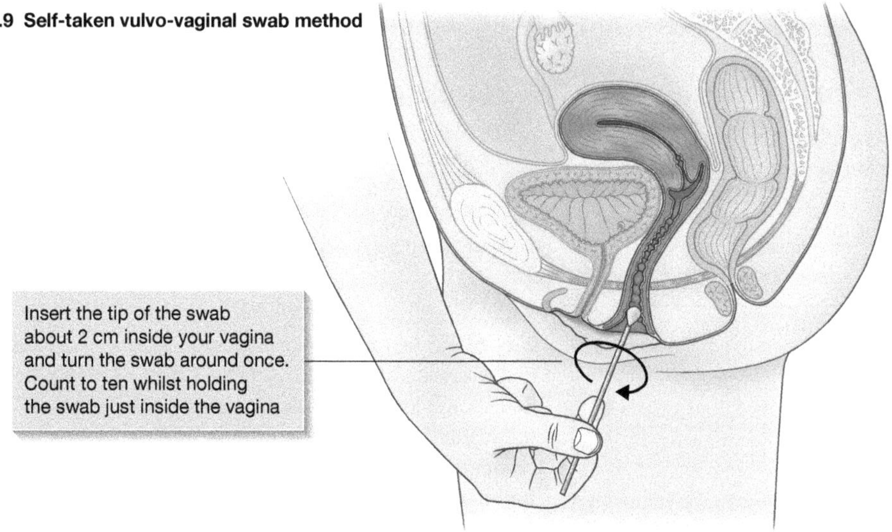

Insert the tip of the swab about 2 cm inside your vagina and turn the swab around once. Count to ten whilst holding the swab just inside the vagina

Table 1.3 Recommended tests and investigations

Clinical situation	Specimen type	Test
Asymptomatic female	Self-taken vulvo-vaginal swab	NAAT for chlamydia and gonorrhoea
	Venous blood sample	Syphilis and HIV
Asymptomatic male	First void urine*	NAAT for chlamydia and gonorrhoea
	Venous blood sample	Syphilis and HIV
Asymptomatic MSM	First void urine* Pharyngeal swab† Rectal swab†	NAAT for chlamydia and gonorrhoea
	Venous blood sample	Syphilis, HIV and hepatitis B Hepatitis C†

* Urine should be held for at least 1 hour before voiding
† If indicated by history/examination

Figure 1.10 Equipment required for an asymptomatic STI screen

General examination

Measurement of BP, weight and height (for body mass index – BMI) is essential in contraceptive consultations. Other systems should be examined depending on the patient's history and the primary purpose of the consultation, for example examining the skin for features of a dermatological disease in a patient complaining of a rash.

Genital examination

The clinical history should indicate the extent of the required examination. For example, a bimanual pelvic examination is not usually indicated unless an aspect of the history raises concerns regarding pelvic pathology. If the patient has symptoms, then a genital examination should be undertaken as follows:

Female examination

• *Inspection of the vulva*: look for discharge, ulcers, blisters, excoriation and inflammation, changes in skin colour or texture and lumps such as genital warts. Noting down negative as well as positive findings will be helpful for future examinations
• Palpate the inguinal region for lymphadenopathy
• *Pass a speculum*: only use a small amount of lubricant such as KY jelly as this can interfere with cervical cytology and measuring the vaginal pH. The speculum can be lubricated with warm water as an alternative
• *Inspect the vagina and cervix*: look for inflammation, a retained foreign body, and assess the amount, colour consistency and odour of any discharge. Document the appearance of the cervix (e.g. healthy, cervical ectropion) and the presence of IUD threads if applicable
• *Bimanual examination*: this should be undertaken only if indicated by the history. Although positive findings such as a mass are helpful, a negative bimanual examination does not exclude pathology (Box 1.8)

Male examination

• Inspection of the anogenital area: look for discharge, skin lesions
• Palpate the inguinal region for lymphadenopathy
• Palpate the scrotal contents for masses and tenderness
• Examine the urethral meatus for discharge and skin lesions

Rectal and oropharyngeal examination

• Should be undertaken in those with symptoms at these sites

Investigations

Specialized SRH services have facilities for on-site microscopy (Figure 1.8). This allows immediate examination and reporting of specimens from patients with symptoms, expediting diagnosis and treatment. Point-of-care tests (POCTs) are also available in some specialist services. It is increasingly common for diagnosis and management of sexually transmitted infections (STIs) to take place

in non-specialist settings such as primary care. New technologies allow less intrusive sampling and facilitate this.

Asymptomatic men and women

• Men and women attending an SRH consultation are often asymptomatic. The development of highly accurate laboratory tests which identify minute amounts of organism DNA and RNA – nucleic acid amplification tests (NAATS) – has enabled the development of self-taken sampling (Figure 1.9)
• These tests do not require viable organisms so are less affected by transport issues, allowing testing to be undertaken in a variety of settings
• The minimum investigations constituting an 'STI screen' in an asymptomatic individual and the method of sampling are listed in Box 1.9, Table 1.3 and Figure 1.10
• An STI screen in an asymptomatic MSM who has had receptive oral sex should include a pharyngeal sample for *Chlamydia trachomatis* and *Neisseria gonorrhoeae* NAATs
• An STI screen in an asymptomatic MSM who has had unprotected receptive anal sex should include a blind rectal sample for *Chlamydia trachomatis* and *Neisseria gonorrhoeae* NAATs

Investigations in symptomatic females

• Vaginal pH: using narrow range pH paper (4–7) (Chapter 12)
• Wet mount and Gram stain: Material from the vaginal walls and posterior vagina can be used to prepare a suspension in normal saline (wet mount) and a Gram-stained smear for immediate microscopy
• High vaginal swab: can be taken in settings without access to immediate microscopy, to transport to the local laboratory
• Endocervical swab: for *Chlamydia trachomatis* and *Neisseria gonorrhoeae* NAAT if the woman is being examined. An additional swab can be taken for microscopy, culture and sensitivity if gonorrhoea is suspected
• Viral swab: for herpes simplex virus and syphilis polymerase chain reaction (PCR) if presenting with anogenital ulcers
• Oropharyngeal and rectal samples for chlamydia and gonorrhoea should be taken in symptomatic patients or high risk situations (e.g. sexual assault)

Investigations in symptomatic males

• *Urethral smear*: on slide for Gram stain (microscopy) and for culture and sensitivity for gonorrhoea
• *First void urine*: for *Chlamydia trachomatis* and *Neisseria gonorrhoeae* NAAT
• *Viral swab*: for herpes simplex virus and syphilis polymerase chain reaction (PCR) if presenting with anogenital ulcers
• *Oropharyngeal and rectal samples* for chlamydia and gonorrhoea NAAT should be taken in symptomatic patients or high risk situations. Additionally, a rectal swab for microscopy (gram stain), culture and sensitivity for gonorrhoea should be taken in men with symptoms of proctitis or anal discharge

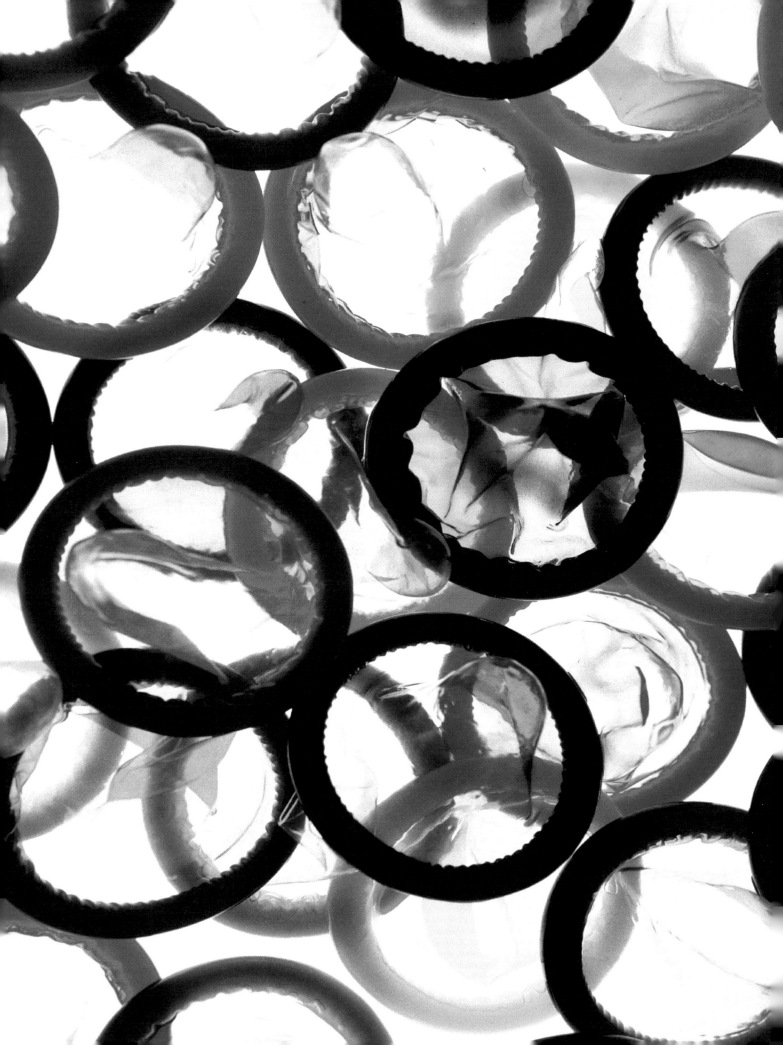

Contraception

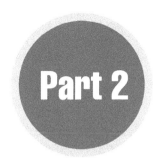

Part 2

Chapters

 Don't forget to visit the companion website at www.ataglanceseries.com/sexualhealth where you can test yourself on these topics.

② # Combined hormonal contraception

Figure 2.1 Primary mechanism of action CHCs

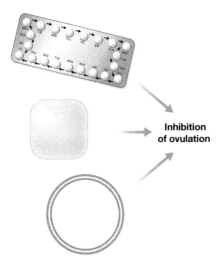

Inhibition of ovulation

Table 2.1 Relative and absolute contraindications to COC for some medical conditions and personal characteristics

Condition	UKMEC 3 (relative contraindication)	UKMEC 4 (absolute contraindication)
BMI	≥ 35 kg/m²	
Smoking and age	Age ≥ 35 years and < 15 cigarettes per day *or* stopped smoking < 1 year ago	Age ≥ 35 years and ≥ 15 cigarettes per day
Hypertension	Adequately controlled *or* systolic > 140 – 159 mmHg *or* diastolic > 90 – 94 mmHg	Systolic ≥ 160 mmHg *or* diastolic ≥ 95 mmHg *or* vascular disease
Stroke		History of cerebrovascular accident or TIA
VTE	Family history of VTE in first-degree relative < 45 years Immobility unrelated to surgery (e.g. acute illness or paralysis)	• History of VTE • Current VTE (on anticoagulants) • Known thrombogenic mutation (e.g. factor V Leiden mutation)
Ischaemic heart disease (IHD)		Current IHD or history of IHD
Headaches	Continuation of CHC if migraine without aura develops during method use at any age	Pre-existing migraine with aura at any age
Breast disease	• Undiagnosed breast mass • Carriers of known gene mutations, e.g. BRCA1 • Past breast cancer with no evidence of recurrence for 5 years	Current breast cancer
Liver disease		Severe cirrhosis Liver adenoma Malignant liver tumours (hepatoma)

Table 2.2 Risk of VTE associated with non-use, CHC use and pregnancy

	Risk of VTE per 10 000 healthy women per year
Non-CHC users and not pregnant	2
CHC users containing EE and:	
• levonorgestrel, norgestimate or norethisterone	5 – 7
• etonogestrel (CVR) or norelgestromin (CTP)	6 – 12
• gestodene, desogestrel or drospirenone	9 – 12
Pregnancy	29
Immediate postpartum	300 – 400

Figure 2.2 Advantages and health benefits of CHC

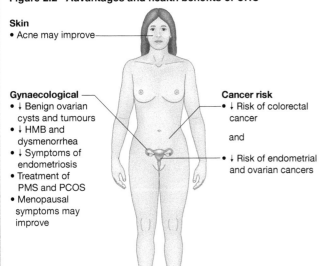

Skin
• Acne may improve

Gynaecological
• ↓ Benign ovarian cysts and tumours
• ↓ HMB and dysmenorrhea
• ↓ Symptoms of endometriosis
• Treatment of PMS and PCOS
• Menopausal symptoms may improve

Cancer risk
• ↓ Risk of colorectal cancer

and

• ↓ Risk of endometrial and ovarian cancers

Figure 2.3 Disadvantages and health risks of CHC

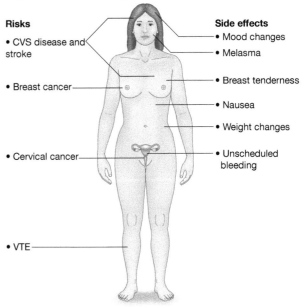

Risks
• CVS disease and stroke
• Breast cancer
• Cervical cancer
• VTE

Side effects
• Mood changes
• Melasma
• Breast tenderness
• Nausea
• Weight changes
• Unscheduled bleeding

Sexual and Reproductive Health at a Glance, First Edition. Catriona Melville. © 2015 by John Wiley & Sons, Ltd. Published 2015 by John Wiley & Sons, Ltd.
Companion website: www.ataglanceseries.com/sexualhealth

Background

Combined hormonal contraceptives (CHCs) are the most commonly used contraceptive methods in the UK and USA. They contain a synthetic estrogen (most commonly ethinylestradiol – EE) and a progestogen (synthetic formulation of progesterone) which can be delivered via the oral ('the pill'), transdermal (contraceptive patch) or vaginal (contraceptive ring) routes.

Mechanism of action

The primary mechanism of action of CHCs is inhibition of ovulation by suppression of LH and FSH via the hypothalamic-pituitary-ovarian axis (Figure 2.1). Secondary effects include alteration of the cervical mucus (thickening) and endometrium (thinning). Seven active continuous days of a CHC method are required to inhibit ovulation and the remainder maintain anovulation.

Efficacy

CHCs are short-acting user-dependent methods so are not as effective at preventing pregnancy as the LARC methods. This is reflected in the typical use failure rate. The combined oral contraceptive pill (COC), combined vaginal ring (CVR) and combined transdermal patch (CTP) were compared in a Cochrane review, which concluded that the methods have similar efficacy:

- perfect use: failure rate is 0.3%
- typical use: failure rate is 9%

Contraindications

The effects of CHCs have been well studied and overall they are very safe. There are, however, women with certain characteristics (e.g. obesity) or with various conditions (e.g. migraine with aura) in which a CHC is not recommended (Table 2.1). For a comprehensive list consult the FRSH UKMEC guidelines (latest version 2009).

Advantages and health benefits (Figure 2.2)

Cancer risk

- **Endometrial and ovarian cancer:** Use of the COC is associated with a reduced risk of ovarian and endometrial cancers. The risk reduces with increased duration of COC use, e.g. after 15 years of use, the risk of these cancers is approximately half those of women who have never used the COC. Although this effect declines over time after stopping, it continues to offer protection for several decades
- **Colorectal cancer:** Current or recent use of the COC is associated with a reduced risk of colorectal cancer

Other benefits

CHC use is associated with many gynaecological benefits. Improvement in acne may occur in some women using CHC methods

Disadvantages and health risks (Figure 2.3)

Venous thromboembolism (VTE)

- CHC use is associated with a small increased risk of VTE compared to non-users
- The risk is highest in the first few months of starting the method
- The absolute risk of VTE is low and returns to normal levels shortly after method discontinuation (within weeks)

- The type of progestogen influences the risk of VTE (Table 2.2) Most women in the UK are therefore started on a COC containing an older progestogen, e.g. levonorgestrel (LNG)
- **Dianette®** contains cyproterone acetate 2 mg and EE 35 μg (this combination is also known as co-cyprindiol). It is indicated for treatment of severe acne and moderate to severe hirsuitism. Use of co-cyprindiol pills is associated with a 1.5–2-fold increased incidence of VTE compared with LNG containing CHCs. Although it has a contraceptive effect it should not be used solely for contraception and should only be used for treatment of acne after topical therapy and systemic antibiotic therapy have failed. Treatment should be withdrawn 3–4 months after the condition has resolved

CVS disease and stroke (Table 2.1)

Some studies have shown a very small increase in absolute risk of MI and stroke in COC users. The risk of MI increases in COC users who smoke and the risk of ischaemic stroke is increased in COC users who have migraine with aura (UKMEC 4). Other factors such as hypertension and obesity also influence risk of vascular disease.

Breast cancer

While a large meta-analysis has shown that current users of the COC have a small increased risk of breast cancer (relative risk 1.24), the risk is not related to duration of use, declines to that of non-users within 10 years of COC cessation, and is not associated with increased mortality from breast cancer.

Cervical cancer

CHC use is associated with a small increase in the risk of cervical cancer, which increases with duration of use and declines with time after stopping.

Mortality

Data from the Royal College of General Practitioners (RCGP) Oral Contraception Study demonstrated that ever-use of COCs was associated with a 12% reduction in all-cause mortality. Other studies show no negative effect on mortality with use of COCs.

Side effects

Minor side effects are often reported with CHC methods but not all have an established causal relationship. They can result in high discontinuation rates, however, so it is important to discuss these with women before initiating the method. Side effects will often resolve within the first 3 months of use. *Unscheduled bleeding* is common (up to 20% of COC users) but this often settles with time. It is important to exclude other causes of bleeding such as missed pills, STIs or pregnancy. *Weight gain*: a causal relationship between CHC methods and weight gain is not supported by existing evidence; however, weight gain is often cited as a reason for discontinuation therefore it is important to address this issue before starting the method. *Breast tenderness* and nausea tend to improve with time. *Melasma* is an acquired hypermelanosis of sun-exposed areas of the face due to exposure to exogenous hormones (estrogen and progestogen). It is precipitated by sun exposure. Avoidance of sunlight is the basis of management however switching to a non-hormonal method may be preferred.

Figure 2.4 Combined transdermal patch (CTP)

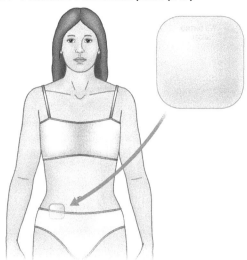

The CTP (Evra® or Ortho Evra®) is a matrix-type transdermal patch with a contact surface area of 20 cm². It releases 33.9 μg of EE and 203 μg of norelgestromin per day.

Administration: One patch is applied to the skin (any clean dry area except the breasts) and changed weekly for 3 consecutive weeks. Following removal of the third patch, there is a patch-free interval of a week during which a withdrawal bleed usually occurs.

Advantages: In some trials CTP users reported better compliance than COC users. Absorption is independent of the the GI system so the CTP provides choice for women with malabsorption resulting from bowel disease.

Disadvantages: CTP users report more breast discomfort, nausea and vomiting and dysmenorrhoea than pill users. It is generally more expensive than the COC.

Figure 2.5 Combined vaginal ring (CVR)

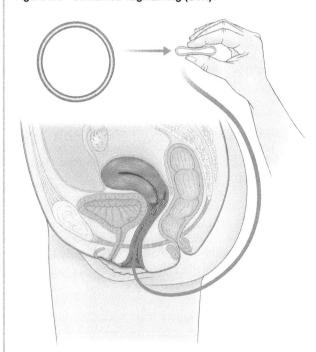

The CVR Nuvaring® is a flexible transparent latex-free ring measuring 4 mm in cross-section and 54 mm in diameter. It is made of ethylene vinylacetate copolymers and magnesium stearate. It delivers 20 μg of etonogestrel and 15 μg of ethinylestradiol per day.

Administration: One ring is inserted into the vagina and left continuously for 3 weeks. It is then removed for 7 days during which time a withdrawal bleed usually occurs. It can be used during sexual intercourse and with tampon use.

Storage: Rings must be stored in a fridge (at 2 – 8°C) until they are dispensed and then can be stored at room temperature for up to 4 months.

Advantages:
• The CVR may offer better cycle control compared with COCs
• Users report less nausea, acne and mood changes than with oral combined methods
• Offers an alternative route of administration for women with malabsorption

Disadvantages:
• More vaginal discharge and irritation is associated with the CVR than other CHCs
• The CVR is generally more expensive than COCs
• Device storage requirements can limit use in some countries

Drug interactions

Hepatic enzyme inducers: Drugs that induce hepatic enzymes increase the metabolism of CHCs, which may reduce their efficacy. Long-term CHC users should therefore switch to a method which is unaffected by these drugs (e.g. an intrauterine method). Short-term users of these drugs (≤2 months) should be advised to use additional precautions for the duration of the course of treatment and for a subsequent 28 days. Consideration can also be given to increasing the dose of EE to at least 50 μg (30 μg is the absolute minimum) and reducing or omitting the pill-free interval. Rifampicin and rifabutin are particularly potent enzyme inducers and therefore women taking these drugs should be advised to switch to a contraceptive method which is unaffected by them (UKMEC 3).

Non-hepatic enzyme inducing antibiotics: The WHOMEC, USMEC (US medical eligibility criteria) and UKMEC advise that non-enzyme-inducing antibiotics can be taken concurrently with CHCs without the need for additional precautions (even for short courses).

Lamotrigine: Concurrent use of CHC can reduce serum concentrations of this anticonvulsant thereby increasing seizure frequency. Serum concentrations of lamotrigine increase on CHC cessation and during the pill free week which can result in an increase in reported side effects and potentially drug toxicity. This effect does not occur when lamotrigine is used in combination with sodium valproate. CHC use with lamotrigine monotherapy is therefore given a UKMEC Category 3.

Ulipristal acetate (UPA): This emergency contraceptive blocks the action of progesterone and could in theory therefore reduce the efficacy of progesterone containing contraceptives. CHC users should take additional contraceptive precautions for 14 days after taking UPA.

Other drugs: Anti-obesity drugs may cause severe diarrhoea or vomiting and therefore could reduce the efficacy of COCs by reducing drug absorption.

Combined oral contraceptives

About a quarter of women in the UK report using 'the pill' and it is well established having been available in the UK and USA for over 50 years. There are a variety of COCs which vary in type of progestogen and dose of estrogen. COCs can either deliver the same dose of progestogen and estrogen in every pill (monophasic/fixed dose pills) or the dose can vary (phasic pills). There is no evidence that phasic pills have any advantages over fixed dose pills. The majority of COCs used in the UK contain 20–35 μg of EE and a progestogen, e.g. levonorgestrel in a fixed dose. **Administration:** Traditionally the COC regimen consists of 21 active pills (1 per day) followed by a 7-day pill-free interval during which a withdrawal bleed occurs due to endometrial shedding. This regimen was designed to mimic the 'natural' menstrual cycle; however, tailored regimens can be used without reducing contraceptive efficacy, e.g. tricycling or continuous CHC use, or reducing the duration of the pill-free interval. Tailored regimens can be used with the CVR and CTP, e.g. continuous use until break-through bleeding occurs. Any alternatives to the standard regimens in the SPC are outwith product licence, however, are endorsed by evidence-based guidelines. **Advantages:** COCs are generally less expensive than other CHC methods and are readily available and easy to use. COCs provide similar cycle control to the CTP. **Disadvantages:** discontinuation of all CHC methods is common. The need for daily dosing may result in poor compliance. **'Natural' estrogen-containing COCs**: *Qlaira*® is a COC containing estradiol valerate (E2V) and dienogest (DNG) in a continuous quadriphasic dosage regimen (26 active tablets and two placebo tablets). Designed to mimic the menstrual cycle's natural hormone changes but evidence of benefit over traditional COCs is limited. It is more expensive than other COCs and has a complex and potentially confusing regimen, with four different missed pill rules.

Zoely® is a monophasic COC containing 17β-estrodiol (as hemihydrate) and nomegestrol acetate (NOMAC). It may have smaller effects on lipid and carbohydrate metabolism than established COCs. It is taken continuously as 24 active followed by four inactive tablets. Withdrawal bleeds are often absent. It is more costly than many established COCs.

Combined transdermal patch

See Figure 2.4.

Combined vaginal ring

See Figure 2.5.

Information for CHC users

Starting regimens

CHC methods containing EE can be started up to day 5 of the menstrual cycle without the need for additional precautions. CHCs can be started at any other time in the menstrual cycle as long as pregnancy risk has been assessed and it is reasonably certain the woman is not pregnant (see Fundamentals Box 1.7). If the method is started after day 5, additional precautions (or abstinence) should be advised for 7 days (7-day rule). EE containing CHC methods can be started on day 21 post partum (non-breastfeeding women) and up to and including day 5 post abortion without the need for additional precautions. Thereafter in both groups of women, the 7-day rule applies.

Advice if CHC has been incorrectly taken

COC: If one pill has been missed (more than 24 hours late) then it should be taken as soon as it is remembered and the pill-taking regimen should continue as usual. Emergency contraception is not required (as long as this is the only missed pill). If two or more consecutive pills have been missed **then** the most recent missed pill should be taken; the remaining pills should be continued; condoms should be used until seven consecutive active pills have been taken. ***Additionally*** if the missed pills are in the first week (pills 1–7) then emergency contraception (EC) should be considered if unprotected sexual intercourse (UPSI) occurred in the pill-free interval. If the pills are missed in the third week (pills 15–21) then the pill-free interval should be omitted by finishing the current pack and starting a new pack the next day. ***CTP and CVR*** if the patch or ring-free interval has been extended by ≤48 hours or the ring or patch has been removed/detached for ≤48 hours then no additional protection is required. >48 hours of ring or patch removal (or increasing the patch/ring free interval by >48 hours) necessitates additional contraceptive precautions and consideration of EC (refer to the MHRA or FSRH for full guidance).

Follow-up

Women should be reviewed 3 months after commencing a CHC method to measure BP and discuss any problems or side effects. Thereafter a 12 months' supply may be offered (3 months of CVR). Women can continue to use a CHC method until 50 years of age provided there are no risk factors which would limit use.

Progestogen-only contraceptives

Table 3.1   POP types available in the UK and USA in 2015

	Progestogen (dose)	Brand name
Traditional POPs	Levonorgestrel (30 µg) Norethisterone (350 µg)	Norgeston® Micronor® Noriday® Nor-QD®
New generation POP	Desogestrel (75 µg)	Cerazette® Cerelle® Nacrez® Aizea®

Table 3.2   Relative and absolute contraindications for the use of PO contraception

Condition	UKMEC category I = initiation; C = continuation		
	POP	PO injectable	PO implant
Multiple risks for CVS disease		3	
Hypertension with vascular disease		3	
Current or history of IHD	3 (C only)	3 (I and C)	3 (C only)
Stroke	3 (C only)	3 (I and C)	3 (C only)
Unexplained vaginal bleeding		3	3
Current breast cancer	4	4	4
Past breast cancer with no evidence of recurrence for 5 years	3	3	3
Diabetes with nephropathy/retinopathy/neuropathy or other vascular disease		3	
Severe (decompensated) cirrhosis	3	3	3
Liver tumours (benign) hepatocellular adenoma	3	3	3
Liver tumours (malignant) hepatoma	3	3	3
Systemic lupus erythematosis (SLE) • Positive (or unknown) antiphospholipid antibodies • Severe thrombocytopenia	3	3 3 (I)	3

Refer to UKMEC 2009 for complete list of conditions and categories

Sexual and Reproductive Health at a Glance, First Edition. Catriona Melville. © 2015 by John Wiley & Sons, Ltd. Published 2015 by John Wiley & Sons, Ltd.
Companion website: www.ataglanceseries.com/sexualhealth

Progestogen-only pills

Background

Progestogen-only pills (POPs) are less commonly used than COCs; they have a good safety profile and can be an extremely valuable option for women in whom the use of estrogen-containing pills (COCs) is either contraindicated or not tolerated. They are often known as the 'mini-pill'. POPs are taken at the same time every day with no pill-free interval.

POP brands available in the UK and USA are listed in Table 3.1. **Mechanism of action:** All POPs alter the cervical mucus, thus preventing penetration of sperm to the upper genital tract. This is the primary mode of action of the 'traditional' POPs. The endometrium is also affected, rendering it unfavourable for implantation. Ovulation is inhibited in up to 60% of cycles with 'traditional' POPs; however, POPs containing the new generation progestogen desogestrel inhibit ovulation in up to 97% of cycles which is their primary mode of action. The cervical mucus changes are fully effective within 48 hours of commencing the method. **Efficacy:** With perfect use, POPs are at least 99% effective in preventing pregnancy. As with all short-acting user-dependent methods, the typical use failure rate will be higher. The efficacy of traditional POPs appears to increase with age and parity (which are usually linked). In a comparative study the desogestrel-containing POP had a lower failure rate than the LNG-containing POP, but this difference was not significant (as the trial had not been powered to detect differences in efficacy). Suboptimal compliance should have less effect on desogestrel-containing POP efficacy because of its primary effect on ovulation. There is no evidence that POP efficacy is reduced in women who weigh >70 kg and therefore the same regimen is used in these women.

Advantages

The POP is a safe method for most women and has far fewer contraindications than estrogen-containing contraception. It is safe in women over 35 years who smoke, have migraine with aura or have known thrombogenic mutations. In younger women, the desogestrel- containing POP has comparable efficacy to the COC, making it a good choice if estrogen is contraindicated. It can be used safely in breastfeeding women and up until the age of 55 years. It is taken as one tablet a day without a pill-free break and this simple regimen may result in better compliance and fewer pill-taking errors.

Disadvantages

Compliance: As with all non-LARC methods, the typical user failure rate is higher than with perfect use. This user-dependent method requires good compliance as POPs must be taken at or within 3 hours of the same time every day. Desogestrel-containing POPs have a '12-hour window' for pill taking. **Contraindications:** Table 3.2 summarizes the conditions which are a relative or absolute contraindication for POP use. (See UKMEC guidance for full categories). **Side effects:** There is *no* evidence of a causal association between the POP and weight change, depression, headache, CVS disease or breast cancer. *Bleeding patterns* changes to bleeding patterns are common with progestogen-only methods and are cited as the most common reason for discontinuation of the POP.

It is important to counsel women about the potential change to their bleeding pattern prior to commencing the method. In general, 20% of women will be amenorrhoeic (this may be viewed as advantageous); 40% will bleed regularly, and 40% will have erratic bleeding. The bleeding is much less predictable than with a combined contraceptive method. **Drug interactions:** Liver enzyme inducing drugs (e.g. phenytoin) increase the metabolism of progestogens and thereby can potentially reduce contraceptive efficacy of POPs. Women taking a short-term course of these drugs should be advised to use condoms in addition to the POP method and for 4 weeks after stopping the course. An alternative contraceptive method is recommended for women on long-term liver enzyme-inducing drug therapy. **Other:** This method does not protect against STIs and condoms should therefore be used in addition if required.

Starting regimens

If the POP is started on days 1–5 of the menstrual cycle it is effective immediately. It can be started at any other time in the menstrual cycle as long as pregnancy risk has been assessed and it is reasonably certain the woman is not pregnant (see Fundamentals Box 1.7). If the method is started after day 5, additional precautions are required for 48 hours. *After induced abortion or miscarriage* the POP should be started immediately or within 5 days. If commenced after this time then additional precautions are required for 48 hours. *Post-partum* initiation can be immediate in both breast- and bottle-feeding women (with no effect on quality or quantity of breast milk). If started more than day 21 postpartum, additional precautions are required for 48 hours.

Missed or late POPs

If a traditional POP is more than 3 hours late (>27 hours have elapsed since the last pill was taken), or a desogestrel-containing POP is taken more than 12 hours late (>36 hours have elapsed since the last pill was taken) then the following missed pill rules apply:

- The missed pill should be taken as soon as it is remembered
- The next pill should be taken at the usual time which may mean taking two pills in 1 day
- Additional precautions are advised for 48 hours (after the POP has been taken)

Emergency contraception may be required if UPSI has occurred in the 48-hour period after the missed pill.

Vomiting

If a woman vomits within 2 hours of taking a POP, then she should take another pill as soon as possible. If she continues to vomit or has severe diarrhoea then the missed pill rules will need to be followed.

Follow-up

Woman may be offered 12 months supply of POP and advised to return for review earlier if there are any problems with the method or changes to her health. *Managing bleeding problems* can be problematic. Other causes for abnormal PVB should be excluded (e.g. STIs and pregnancy). Changing the type or dose of progestogen may help but if this an unacceptable bleeding pattern persists then an alternative method may need to be considered.

Table 3.3 Progestogen-only injectables in the UK

Drug name	Progestogen type and dose	Administration
Depo-provera®	Depot medroxyprogesterone acetate (DMPA) 150 mg	12 weekly (SPC), 13 weekly (FSRH, out with licence) by deep intramuscular (IM) injection
Sayana Press®	Depot medroxyprogesterone acetate (DMPA) 104 mg	13 weeks (± 7 days) by subcutaneous (SC) injection
Noristerat®	Norethisterone enantate (NET-EN) 200 mg	8 weeks by deep IM injection: only licenced for short-term use

Box 3.1 Risk factors for osteoporosis

- Immobility
- Poor diet
- Smoking
- Alcohol
- Family history
- Use of high dose steroids
- Medical conditions, e.g. thyroid disease, Crohn's disease

Box 3.2 Lifestyle advice for bone protection

Advice to users of DMPA:

- Undertake regular weight-bearing exercise
- Eat a balanced diet containing calcium and Vitamin D, e.g. oily fish
- Advise smoking cessation
- Advise alcohol intake within recommended limits

Figure 3.1 Sayana Press

Background

- Launched in the UK in 2013 (also available in the USA)
- Subcutaneous (SC) DMPA delivered via Uniject delivery system
- Efficacy, return to fertility, weight gain and BMD effects similar to IM DMPA
- Injection site reactions are more common with SC than with IM DMPA

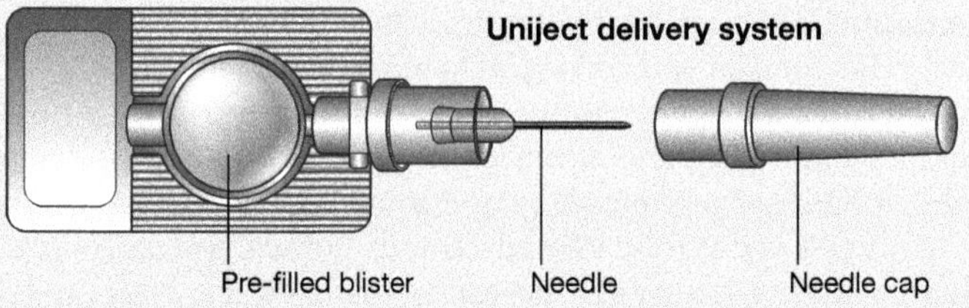

Uniject delivery system

Pre-filled blister   Needle   Needle cap

Benefits of SC administration

- May facilitate self-administration, however, this is currently not licensed
- May be less likely to cause haematoma than IM injection (e.g. in women taking anticoagulants, or with bleeding disorders)
- May be advantageous in very obese women (where there is difficulty in reaching muscle for IM injection)

Box 3.3 Bridging methods

- If the contraceptive method of choice cannot be started immediately then a short-acting method, e.g. CHC, POP, can be used temporarily until pregnancy is excluded and a longer-acting method can be initiated
- Bridging methods can also be used when pregnancy has been excluded but the method of choice is not immediately available

Figure 3.2 Management of late or missed progestogen-only injection

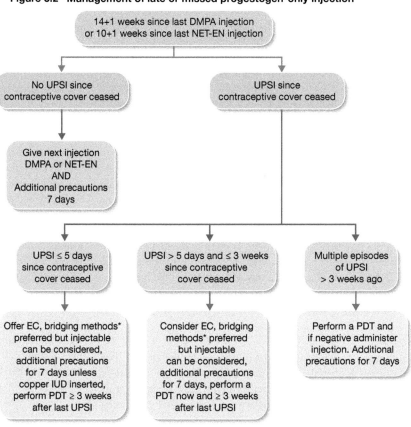

14+1 weeks since last DMPA injection or 10+1 weeks since last NET-EN injection

No UPSI since contraceptive cover ceased

Give next injection DMPA or NET-EN AND Additional precautions 7 days

UPSI since contraceptive cover ceased

UPSI ≤ 5 days since contraceptive cover ceased

Offer EC, bridging methods* preferred but injectable can be considered, additional precautions for 7 days unless copper IUD inserted, perform PDT ≥ 3 weeks after last UPSI

UPSI > 5 days and ≤ 3 weeks since contraceptive cover ceased

Consider EC, bridging methods* preferred but injectable can be considered, additional precautions for 7 days, perform a PDT now and ≥ 3 weeks after last UPSI

Multiple episodes of UPSI > 3 weeks ago

Perform a PDT and if negative administer injection. Additional precautions for 7 days

*Bridging methods see Box 3.3

Progestogen-only injectable contraception

Background

There are three progestogen-only (PO) injectable contraceptives available in the UK (Table 3.3). Intramuscular (IM) DMPA (Depo-Provera®) is most commonly used however a subcutaneous (SC) formulation of medroxyprogesterone acetate (DMPA) was launched in 2013 (Sayana Press®). Data from the Office of National Statistics Opinions Survey Report on contraception showed that 3% of women in Great Britain aged 16–49 years used injectable contraception in 2008/2009. This figure has remained fairly static for the past 5 years. **Mode of action:** Progestogen-only injectable contraception works primarily by inhibition of ovulation. Secondary effects include thickening of the cervical mucus and alteration of the endometrium rendering it unfavourable for implantation. **Efficacy:** Progestogen-only injectable contraceptives are LARC methods and therefore have superior efficacy to short acting methods. If given within the recommended dosing interval then the failure rate is approximately 0.2% in the first year of use. With typical use the failure rate approximates 6%. **Dose:** See Table 3.3. **Administration:** DMPA is a sterile aqueous suspension generally in a pre-filled syringe. Both SC and IM formulations must be vigorously shaken just before use to ensure complete suspension of the contents. It should be given by deep intramuscular injection preferably into the gluteus maximus muscle. An alternative site is the deltoid. NET-EN is an oily solution with high viscosity at low temperatures; therefore, it is suggested that the vial is submersed in warm water before use. Sayana Press® is given subcutaneously into the upper anterior thigh or the abdomen (Figure 3.1).

Advantages

DMPA is a safe contraceptive choice for most women with the only absolute contraindication being current breast cancer (UKMEC4). For relative contraindications see Table 3.2. It can be used in women in whom the use of estrogen-containing methods is contraindicated. As it is a long-acting method its efficacy does not depend on daily administration. It inhibits ovulation and may reduce the symptoms of PMS and endometriosis and reduce dysmenorrhoea. **Drug interactions:** The efficacy of DMPA is unaffected by either antibiotics or liver enzyme-inducing drugs. **Health effects:** A causal association with method use and VTE has not been demonstrated. There is insufficient evidence to verify or disprove an association with MI or stroke. There may be a weak association between current use of a PO- injectable and a (probably small) risk of breast cancer. This is likely to reduce with time after stopping.

Disadvantages

Side effects: *Weight gain* DMPA use is associated with weight gain. On average women will gain 3 kg by 2 years of use (range 2–6.1 kg). There is evidence that adolescent women (aged <18 years) with a higher BMI at initiation of the method (≥ 30 kg/m^2) are likely to gain more weight during DMPA use than those with a lower BMI (<25) at initiation. *Changes to bleeding pattern* Altered bleeding patterns are common with DMPA use. About half of women will be amenorrhoeic by 1 year and 70% by 2 years of use. This may be viewed positively by women. Other bleeding patterns including infrequent bleeding, spotting or prolonged bleeding may be less acceptable than amenorrhoea resulting in discontinuation of the method. *Other side effects* Acne, mood changes, reduced libido, headaches, vaginitis and alopecia have all been cited as side effects of DMPA however there is little available evidence to demonstrate causation. **Bone mineral density (BMD):** The influence of DMPA on bone density has caused controversy in some countries, most notably the USA where the FDA added a 'black box warning' to the labelling of Depo-provera in 2004. Concerns are based on the premise that DMPA lowers estradiol levels (due to inhibition of follicular development), which in theory can cause a reduction in BMD. Evidence to date suggests that current use of DMPA is associated with a small reduction in BMD, which is usually regained on method cessation. It is unclear whether this translates to an increased risk of fracture. There is some concern about the impact of DMPA on BMD in adolescents as it causes a reduction in BMD at a time when they have not yet achieved their peak bone mass, and BMD is normally increasing. Because of these concerns, it is recommended that DMPA is only used in women <18 years after other options have been considered. Nonetheless, it is still a common choice in women of this age group. The FSRH and MRHA advise that women using DMPA should be reviewed every 2 years taking into account the individuals risk factors for osteoporosis (Boxes 3.1 and 3.2). If significant risk factors are established, then alternative contraception should be considered. **Return to fertility:** Ovulation can be delayed by up to 1 year after discontinuation of the progestogen-only injectable; however, there is no evidence of reduced fertility in the longer term.

Starting regimens

If DMPA is initiated on days 1–5 of a normal menstrual cycle then no additional precautions are required. It can be initiated at any other time in the menstrual cycle as long as pregnancy risk has been assessed and it is reasonably certain the woman is not pregnant (see Fundamentals Box 1.7). If the method is started after day 5, additional precautions are required for 7 days. *After induced abortion or miscarriage* DMPA should be started immediately or within 5 days. If commenced after day 5 then additional precautions are required for 7 days. *Postpartum* initiation can be immediate in bottle feeding women and the method can be used without restriction. In breastfeeding women the SPC for IM DMPA recommends that initiation of the method should be delayed until at least 6 weeks postpartum. DMPA can be used safely by breastfeeding women and the FSRH recommends that initiation under 6 weeks outweighs any potential risks (UKMEC category 2) although ideally it should be delayed until day 21. If started after day 21 postpartum then additional precautions are required for 7 days (breastfeeding and non-breastfeeding women).

Missed or late injections (Figure 3.2)

The SPC for IM DMPA advises a 12 weekly dosing interval (13 weeks for SC DMPA , 8 weeks for NET-EN). The FSRH recommends giving repeat IM DMPA at 13 weekly intervals (out with product licence) to provide consistency with the SC DMPA regimen. A repeat injection can be given late (up to 14 weeks since last injection for IM and SC DMPA or 10 weeks for NET-EN) without additional precautions as the risk of ovulation is low.

Follow-up

Review at the time of each injection and note any changes to the medical history or the development of any side effects. Continuation of the method should be reviewed on a 2-yearly basis.

Bleeding problems: If other causes of bleeding, e.g. STIs are, excluded then reassurance may suffice as the bleeding pattern will often settle with further injections. There is some evidence that EE (as a COC) or mefenamic acid can be helpful in managing unacceptable bleeding associated with this method.

Box 3.4 ENG implant insertion

Insertion site:
Insert implant subdermally in the inner side of the upper arm 8 – 10 cm above the medial epicondyle of the humerus. Insert just under the skin to avoid the neurovascular bundle which lies between the biceps and triceps muscle (Figures 3.2 and 3.3).

Procedure:
• HCP should be seated to directly visualise the needle tip as it punctures the skin
• Mark the arm at both the insertion site and 6 – 8cm above this to guide the direction of the implant
• Aseptic hand hygiene and sterile gloves should be used
• Clean insertion site with antiseptic solution
• Inject the insertion site and 'insertion tunnel' with local anaesthesia (e.g. 2 mL of 1% lidocaine)
• Puncture the skin with the applicator needle tip with the applicator at an angle of about 30° then lower the applicator until it is in a horizontal position
• Advance the needle to its full length while tenting the skin
• Unlock the purple slider (Figure 3.3) by pushing it slightly downwards and then fully backwards until it stops. This releases the implant, leaving it in its subdermal position
• The needle is now safely locked inside the applicator which can be removed
• The HCP and preferably the woman should palpate the implant immediately after insertion to confirm it is present. This should be documented
• Close the skin with a small adhesive dressing ± a gauze bandage to minimize bruising
• Give wound care instructions and implant user card with the service contact details
• No routine follow-up is required unless problems arise or there is a change to the medical history

Box 3.5 ENG implant removal

• Examine the arm to ensure the implant is palpable
• Mark the distal end of the implant (nearest the elbow)
• Use an aseptic technique and anaesthetize the removal site
• Whilst pushing on the proximal end of the implant make a small longitudinal incision (approx. 2 mm) over the distal end of the implant
• Push the implant gently towards the incision until the tip is visible
• Grasp the tip with forceps and remove the implant
• If the implant does not become visible in the incision, the forceps are gently inserted into the incision and the implant grasped
• If the implant is encapsulated then a small incision is made into the tissue sheath before removal and the tissue around the implant can then be carefully dissected before grasping the implant with a second pair of forceps
• Confirm that the device has been removed in its entirety
• Close the skin incision with a steri-strip ± a gauze bandage to minimize bruising

Box 3.6 Replacing an ENG implant

• An implant can be immediately replaced after removal of the previous implant
• This can be in the same arm and via the same incision but along a fresh track adjacent to the previous track
• After 2 consecutive implants in the same arm, consider swapping arms (theoretical risk of skin atrophy)
• If the change is within 3 years (or the licensed duration) of insertion of the existing device, then there is no need for additional precautions either before or after the procedure
• If an implant is removed and an alternative method of contraception is started immediately then no additional contraceptive precautions are necessary

Figure 3.3 Cross-sectional anatomy of the upper arm

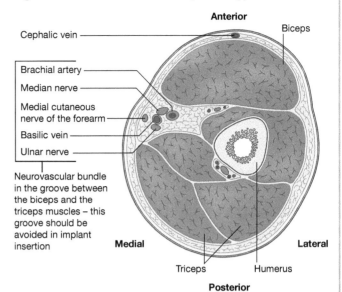

Neurovascular bundle in the groove between the biceps and the triceps muscles – this groove should be avoided in implant insertion

Figure 3.4 Site of implant insertion

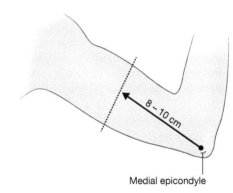

Figure 3.5 Nexplanon applicator

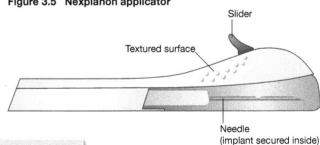

Progestogen-only implants

Background

Nexplanon® (USA and UK) is a single subdermal rod licensed for 3 years' use. In Australia it is marketed as Implanon NXT®. It differs only from its predecessor Implanon in that it is radio-opaque, and has a different insertion technique and application device. Other subdermal contraceptive implants available worldwide include Norplant® and Jadelle®. Norplant®, a six-rod LNG implant is no longer available in the USA, the UK and most Western countries; however, it is still used in the developing world. Jadelle – a two-rod LNG implant – has succeeded Norplant in countries such as New Zealand. Both Jadelle and Norplant are licensed for 5 years' continuous use. **Nexplanon** (Implanon NXT) is a soft flexible rod containing 68 mg of etonogestrel (ENG) within an ethylene vinylacetate copolymer. It is 4 cm long and 2 mm in diameter and non-biodegradable. The release rate of ENG reduces over time from approximately 60–70 μg/day in weeks 5–6 post insertion to 35–45 μg/day at the end of the first year. *Mechanism of action* Inhibition of ovulation is the primary mode of action. Additionally the progestogen-only implant (in common with other progestogen-only contraceptives) alters the cervical mucus thus preventing penetration of sperm to the upper genital tract. The endometrium is also affected rendering it unfavourable for implantation. *Efficacy* The progestogen-only implant is a LARC and is therefore highly efficacious. NICE reports the overall pregnancy rate over 3 years of use as <1 in 1000. True failures of this method are rare with reported pregnancies often the result of drug interactions or incorrect timing of insertion. There is an inverse relationship between weight and serum etonogestrel levels. However no increased pregnancy risk has been demonstrated in women weighing up to 149 kg but the manufacturer states that earlier replacement can be considered in 'heavier' women (although does not define what BMI or weight this constitutes). There is no direct evidence to support earlier replacement.

Advantages

This highly efficacious estrogen-free method can be used safely in most women. **Gynaecological:** It may reduce dysmenorrhoea and symptoms of endometriosis in some women and 20% of users will have amenorrhoea while using this method which some will find advantageous. **Fertility:** There is no delay in return to fertility on discontinuation of this method. **Compliance:** As this method does not depend on daily or frequent administration it is a good choice for women who are forgetful at using other methods. **Changes to weight, mood or libido:** There is no evidence of a causal relationship between the progestogen-only implant and weight change, mood change or reduction in libido.

Health effects

There is no association with an increased risk of stroke or MI and little or no increased risk of VTE with progestogen-only implants. There is a lack of robust evidence concerning the impact of progestogen-only implants on breast cancer risk; however, any attributable risk – if present at all – is likely to be very small. Although a reduction in BMD may be seen with this method, there is no evidence of a clinically significant effect.

Disadvantages

Side effects *Contraindications* The only absolute contraindication to use of a progestogen-only implant is current breast cancer (UKMEC 4). There are few relative contraindications (UKMEC 3), which are listed in Table 3.2. *Change to bleeding patterns* Alteration to bleeding patterns is common with this method and is the most frequent reason given for early discontinuation. Approximately 20% of users will have amenorrhoea, while up to 50% will have infrequent, frequent or prolonged bleeding. The problematic bleeding patterns with this method are not likely to settle with time. *Acne* may occur, improve or worsen whilst using this method. *Drug interactions* The efficacy of progestogen-only implants is reduced by concurrent use of liver enzyme inducing drugs (e.g. some anticonvulsants). Non-enzyme inducing antibiotics do not affect the efficacy of this method. Additional precautions i.e. barrier methods should be used with the method if a short course (<3 weeks) of an enzyme-inducing drug is taken and for 4 weeks after the drug has stopped. An alternative contraceptive method should be considered for women on long-term liver enzyme inducing drug therapy.

Starting regimens

The progestogen-only implant can be inserted on days 1–5 of the menstrual cycle without the need for additional precautions. It can also be inserted at any other time in the menstrual cycle if an assessment of pregnancy risk has been made and the clinician is reasonably certain that the women is not pregnant (see Fundamentals Box 1.7). If the method is started after day 5, additional precautions are required for 7 days. *After induced abortion or miscarriage* the progestogen-only implant should be started immediately or within 5 days. If commenced after day 5 then additional precautions are required for 7 days. *Postpartum* The SPC for Nexplanon recommends initiation between days 21 and 28 post partum; however, a progestogen-only implant can be inserted before and up to day 21 postpartum without the need for additional precautions (out with product licence). If a progestogen-only implant is inserted after day 21 postpartum then additional precautions are required for 7 days. The method does not affect the composition or quantity of breast milk and there are no restrictions in use for breastfeeding women.

Insertion and removal techniques for ENG implants (Figures 3.3–3.5, Boxes 3.4–3.5)

The device should be inserted and removed by a healthcare professional (HCP) with appropriate training. Emergency equipment should be available in settings where insertion or removal procedures are performed. For implant replacement see Box 3.6.

Management of complications

Complications with removal. Potential complications including impalpable or broken implants or implant migration are uncommon, particularly since Implanon was replaced by its successor Nexplanon. The device applicator was designed to minimize the risk of deep and non- insertions which resulted in an implant being impalpable at the time of removal. Although Nexplanon can be visualized by X-ray or computed tomography (CT) scan, the first line imaging technique for localization of an impalpable device remains linear array ultrasound. Once the device has been localized by imaging, removal should be undertaken by an expert. Ultrasound guidance may be used for this. **Management of bleeding problems.** Women presenting with a persistent change to their bleeding pattern should be assessed for other possible causes, e.g. STIs. There is a lack of evidence regarding the efficacy of treatments for bleeding problems with ENG implants and most evidence is extrapolated from LNG implants. If other pathology is excluded or treated and the problem persists, a COC can be given (if eligible) for 3 months either cyclically or continuously (outside product license). In the longer term, if the bleeding pattern remains unacceptable then an alternative contraceptive method may need to be considered.

Table 4.1 Common conditions or circumstances where the Cu-IUD or LNG-IUS may be relatively (UKMEC 3) or absolutely (UKMEC 4) contraindicated

Condition	Cu-IUD	LNG-IUS
Postpartum • Between 48 hours and 4 weeks postpartum • Puerperal sepsis	UKMEC 3 UKMEC 4	UKMEC 3 UKMEC 4
Post abortion • Immediately post-septic abortion	UKMEC 4	UKMEC 4
Current and history of ischaemic heart disease	UKMEC 1	UKMEC 2 (initiation) UKMEC 3 (continuation)
Stroke (history of cerebrovascular accident or TIA)	UKMEC 1	UKMEC 2 (initiation) UKMEC 3 (continuation)
Unexplained vaginal bleeding (suspicious) before evaluation	UKMEC 4	UKMEC 4
Gestational trophoblastic disease • Persistently elevated β-hCG levels or malignant disease	UKMEC 4	UKMEC 4
Cervical cancer (awaiting treatment)	UKMEC 4 (initiation) UKMEC 2 (continuation)	UKMEC 4 (initiation) UKMEC 2 (continuation)
Breast cancer • Current • Past and no evidence of current disease for 5 years	UKMEC 1 UKMEC 1	UKMEC 4 UKMEC 3
Distortion of the uterine cavity due to uterine fibroids or any congenital or acquired uterine abnormality that is incompatible with IUD insertion	UKMEC 3	UKMEC 3
Current PID	UKMEC 4 (initiation) UKMEC 2 (continuation)	UKMEC 4 (initiation) UKMEC 2 (continuation)
STIs: symptomatic or asymptomatic chlamydial infection; current purulent cervicitis or gonorrhoea	UKMEC 4 (initiation) UKMEC 2 (continuation)	UKMEC 4 (initiation) UKMEC 2 (continuation)
Liver disease • Severe (decompensated cirrhosis) • Hepatocellular liver tumour (adenoma) • Hepatoma (malignant)	UKMEC 1	UKMEC 3
Systemic lupus erythematosus (SLE) • Positive (or unknown) antiphospholipid antibodies • Severe thrombocytopenia	UKMEC 1 UKMEC 3 (initiation) UKMEC 2 (continuation)	UKMEC 3 UKMEC 2

Figure 4.5 Sounding the uterus

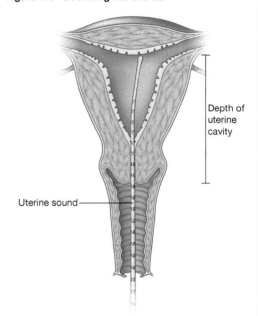

Depth of uterine cavity

Uterine sound

Figure 4.6 Fundal placement of device

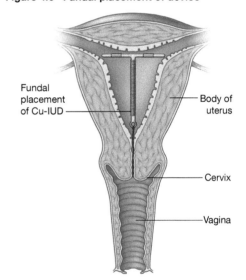

Fundal placement of Cu-IUD

Body of uterus

Cervix

Vagina

Figure 4.7 Lost threads: causes

Correctly located device: threads are drawn up or short

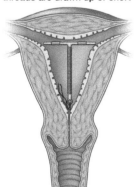

Expulsion: device has been expelled from the uterus

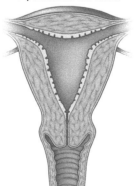

Perforation: device is in an extrauterine location

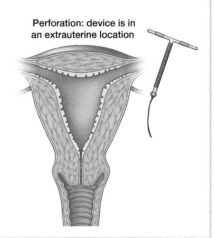

- **Perforation** of the uterus is rare, occurring in less than two per 1000 insertions. The expertise of the clinician inserting the device may influence the rate of perforation
- **Pelvic infection** rates are increased sixfold in the first 20 days following intrauterine device insertion however the overall risk is low. Infection is thought to be due to the introduction of organisms into the uterus at the time of insertion. The risk is related to the background risk of STIs. Women at higher risk of STIs (see Fundamentals Box 1.7) should be offered screening prior to insertion of intrauterine contraception and if results of the STI screen are unavailable before the procedure then antibiotic prophylaxis should be considered. A regimen effective against *C. trachomatis* and *N. Gonorrhoeae* (depending on local prevalence) should be used. Insertion should be delayed in women with symptomatic pelvic infection until they have been treated and the symptoms have resolved. Although transient bacteraemia has been identified during intrauterine contraception procedures, NICE recommends that prophylactic antibiotics to protect against bacterial endocarditis are **not** indicated for insertion or removal of intrauterine contraception even in women with conditions where the risk of infective endocarditis may be increased (e.g. heart valve replacement, previous infective endocarditis)

Contraindications (Table 4.1)
Insertion procedure

General requirements: Insertion should take place in a setting where emergency equipment is accessible and an assistant available throughout the procedure to help should an emergency arise. All staff should be trained in basic life support. The HCP undertaking the procedure should be appropriately trained. Pain relief, e.g. intracervical anaesthesia, should be available and discussed in advance of insertion.

Timing of insertion: A Cu-IUD or LNG-IUS can be inserted at any time during the menstrual cycle if an assessment of pregnancy risk has been made and the clinician is reasonably certain that the women is not pregnant (see Fundamentals Box 1.7). The Cu-IUD is immediately effective for contraception, however the LNG-IUS requires additional precautions for 7 days if inserted out with days 1–7 of the menstrual cycle. If UPSI has occurred prior to insertion, the Cu-IUD can still be inserted as long as this is carried out prior to implantation, i.e. it is inserted up to 5 days after the earliest predicted date of ovulation, or up to 5 days after the first episode of UPSI. The LNG-IUS cannot be inserted in these circumstances as it takes 7 days to become effective. ***After induced abortion, miscarriage or postpartum:*** intrauterine contraception should ideally be inserted at the time or within the first 48 hours after a pregnancy or delayed until 4 or more weeks to reduce the risk of perforation. Insertion between 48 hours and 4 weeks post abortion by an experienced clinician may be the best option to reduce the risk of a subsequent unplanned pregnancy. ***Postpartum:*** the earliest predicted date of ovulation postpartum is thought to be day 28 and therefore a Cu-IUD inserted at this time requires no additional precautions. Insertion of an LNG-IUS from day 28 postpartum onwards will necessitate additional precautions or abstinence for 7 days. There are no restrictions in use of intrauterine contraceptive methods for breastfeeding women.

Insertion technique: There is no evidence to support cleansing of the ectocervix prior to the procedure, and sterile gloves are not required if a 'no-touch' technique is employed (i.e. anything which is to be inserted into the uterine cavity is held only by the handle). Following bimanual examination to assess the size, mobility, position and shape of the uterus, a single-toothed tenaculum or similar forceps should be applied to the cervix to stabilize the uterus. The uterus should be sounded to assess the length of the cavity (Figure 4.5). This will reduce the risk of perforation and ensure fundal placement of the device (Figure 4.6). The device should be inserted according to manufacturer's instructions and the threads trimmed. The woman should be given a record of the type of device inserted (including duration of use), and the arrangements for follow-up. Women can be shown how to check the threads of their intrauterine contraceptive device, and should be told to seek advice and use additional precautions if the threads are not present or the stem of the device is palpable.

Follow-up: Women should be offered a follow-up appointment 3-6 weeks following device insertion. An examination at this time will exclude perforation, infection and expulsion of the device. Women should be told to attend at any subsequent time should they have any concerns regarding the method; however, routine annual check-ups are not indicted.

Removal of intrauterine contraception

An intrauterine device can be removed at any time in the menstrual cycle if pregnancy is planned. Fertility is immediately restored following removal of intrauterine contraception so in order to avoid pregnancy the woman should be advised to abstain from SI or use a barrier method for the 7 days prior to removal of the device. Alternatively, the device can be removed in the first few days of the menstrual cycle. If pregnancy is planned pre-conceptual advice should be given.

Management of lost IUD threads

If the threads of the uterine device cannot be seen on examination, there are three possible causes (Figure 4.7):

1 Correctly located device: the device is in the correct location and the threads are either short or have been drawn into the uterine cavity.
2 Expulsion: the device has been expelled from the uterine cavity.
3 Perforation: the device has perforated and is in an extrauterine location.

Pregnancy should be excluded, additional precautions advised, and an ultrasound scan should be arranged to locate the device. If it is not seen in the uterine cavity then a plain abdominal X-ray should be requested to look for an extrauterine location. If the device is not seen on ultrasound scan or X-ray it can be safely assumed that it has been expelled. If the ultrasound scan shows the correct intrauterine location of the device then the woman can be reassured and the device retained for contraception.

Presence of actinomyces-like organisms (ALO)

Actinomyces israelii is a genital tract commensal which can sometimes be identified on swabs. There is no need to remove intrauterine contraception if ALO is found in an asymptomatic woman.

⑤ Barrier methods

Box 5.1 Male condom checklist

- Store condoms in a cool dry place
- Check kite mark (or other quality certification symbol)
- Check expiry date
- Use a new condom for each episode of sex
- Use only one condom at a time
- Take care not to tear condom when opening (e.g. with sharp nails or teeth)
- Put condom on the penis before any genital contact and only when the penis is erect
- Squeeze tip to expel air and roll condom down to base of penis
- If attempt is made to put condom on inside out then discard condom and use a fresh one
- Only use water soluble lubricants with latex condoms and do not put lubricant inside the condom
- Withdraw the penis after ejaculation (before penis becomes soft) whilst holding condom at the base
- Remove the condom away from the genital area
- Check the condom for tears or breakages
- Wrap the condom and dispose of in the bin

Figure 5.1 Female condom in the vagina

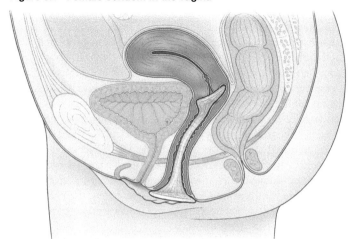

Figure 5.2 Types of diaphragm

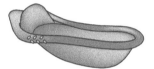

Caya® single size diaphragm

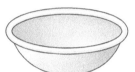

Coil spring

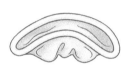

Arcing spring
(option if cervix in difficult position)

Figure 5.3 Femcap

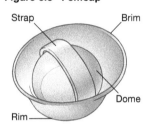

Strap · Brim · Dome · Rim

Table 5.1 Medical conditions given a UKMEC category 3 for use of diaphragms and caps

Medical condition	Comment
HIV infected or high risk of HIV (both using ART and not using ART)	These methods require the use of a spermicide and the only spermicide widely available in the UK is N-9, which can be associated with the development of genital lesions - may increase the risk of HIV acquisition
History of toxic shock syndrome (TSS)	Methods are associated with an increased risk of non-menstrual TSS
Sensitivity to latex proteins (applies to latex diaphragms only)	Use silicone or non-latex barrier method

Additional precautions
• The cap should not be used in women with CIN or cervical cancer
• Diaphragms and caps are not suitable for women who are less than 6 weeks postpartum
• These methods should not be used when menstruating due to the risk of TSS

Box 5.2 Sources of male and female condom failure

- Non-use
- Incorrect storage
- Put on too late/ after genital contact has occurred
- Removed too late
- Condom breaks or tears (associated with wrong lubricant, ill-fitting condoms, increased length of intercourse)
- Condom slips off during sex

Table 5.2 Advantages and disadvantages of barrier methods

Advantages of barrier methods
• No serious side-effects
• Diaphragm or cap can be inserted before sex and use is under woman's control
• Condoms offer STI protection in addition to contraception

Disadvantages of barrier methods
• Contraceptive failure rate is higher than with some of the other available methods
• Spermicide used with diaphragms and caps can be messy and cause irritation
• Chemicals in latex barrier methods can cause irritation in the user or partner
• Users may have difficulty inserting or removing diaphragms and caps
• Users may find condom use interrupts spontaneity during sex
• Some vaginal or topical drugs can damage latex barrier methods (Box 5.3)
• Diaphragm use has been linked to urinary tract infection due to pressure on the urethra. Changing to a slightly smaller or softer device may alleviate this

Box 5.3 Examples of vaginal and topical drugs which may damage latex barrier methods

Clotrimazole

Econazole

Fenticonazole

Isoconazole

Miconazole

Sexual and Reproductive Health at a Glance, First Edition. Catriona Melville. © 2015 by John Wiley & Sons, Ltd. Published 2015 by John Wiley & Sons, Ltd.
Companion website: www.ataglanceseries.com/sexualhealth

Background

Barrier methods are indicated for contraception and may also reduce or prevent the transmission of some STIs. Types of barrier methods available include male and female condoms, diaphragms and cervical caps. They are available in different materials including latex, nitrile, silicone and polyurethane. Barrier methods are user dependent and their efficacy therefore depends on typical use and the background fertility rate. Dams (sometimes know as dental dams) are latex or polyurethane squares of material which act as a barrier between the mouth and anus or mouth and female genitals during oral sexual contact. They are not contraceptive but can prevent transmission of STIs.

Male and female condoms

Mode of action These methods act as a barrier to physically prevent semen entering the body and to prevent contact with the cervicovaginal secretions. They can be used in addition to other contraceptive methods or as a standalone method. **Guidance for use:** Box 5.1 lists the key points, which can be incorporated into a condom demonstration. Female condoms are lubricated sheaths which are inserted into the vagina. They have a ring or sponge at the closed end, which is inserted into the vagina and holds it in place. The open end of the sheath has a larger ring or a flexible frame and remains outside the vagina during sexual intercourse (Figure 5.1). **Contraceptive efficacy:** Condoms are user-dependent methods and as such the efficacy depends on correct and consistent use of the method (Box 5.2).

Perfect use (efficacy)	Typical use
Male condom: 98% effective	82% effective
Female condom: 95% effective	79% effective

Non-latex male condoms have higher clinical breakage rates than latex male condoms, but the pregnancy rates are similar for both types.

STI prevention: Consistent and correct use of latex male condoms is recommended to reduce the risk of sexual transmission of HIV and hepatitis B and C as well as other STIs including *Chlamydia trachomatis*, *Neisseria gonorrhoeae*, *Trichomonas vaginalis* and syphilis. There is conflicting evidence regarding the benefits of condoms in preventing transmission of HPV and herpes simplex viruses as these infections can be transmitted by direct contact with infected skin or mucosal areas not covered by a condom. Nonetheless it is recommended that if used consistently and correctly, male latex condoms may reduce the risk of transmission of these infections. Additionally there is some evidence to support an increase in the rate of HPV clearance and CIN regression when male latex condoms are used correctly. Studies suggest that female and non-latex male condoms offer similar protection to the male latex condom.

Lubricant and spermicide: Most male and female condoms are pre-lubricated. Additional lubricant can be used; however, care must be taken with latex condoms as oil-based products, e.g. body oils, petroleum jelly, can damage latex and increase the risk of condom breakage. The WHO no longer recommends spermicide-lubricated condoms as there is no evidence that they provide any additional protection (against pregnancy and STIs) compared with non-spermicide-lubricated condoms and there are concerns that nonoxinol-9 (the main spermicide available in the UK) is associated with an increased risk of genital lesions due to cell membrane disruption. Lubricant should not be applied inside the condom (gel charging) as this increases the risk of condom slippage. **Anal sex:** Non-oil-based lubricant should be applied inside the anus and over the outside of the condom before anal sex as this reduces the incidence of condom breakage. Contrary to former guidance, evidence demonstrates that thicker condoms (e.g. extra strong or ultra strong) do not confer any advantages over standard condoms in terms of condom breakage or slippage during anal sex. Female condoms may be used for anal sex (with the ring at the end removed). **Contraindications:** A UKMEC category 3 (relative contraindication) is given to users of latex condoms in individuals with a sensitivity to latex proteins.

Diaphragms and caps

Mode of action These methods are used with spermicide and cover the cervix providing a physical and chemical barrier to sperm. **Contraceptive efficacy:** The effectiveness of diaphragms and caps in preventing pregnancy is estimated at between 92% and 96% depending on correct and consistent use with spermicide.

Types of devices

Diaphragms are thin dome-shaped devices made from latex or silicone which cover the cervix, lying across the vagina from the posterior fornix to behind the pubic bone. The Reflexions® flat spring diaphragm was recently discontinued leaving 3 main options in the UK (Figure 5.2). Diaphragms are available in diameters ranging from 55 to 95 mm in 5-mm increments. **Caya®** (formerly known as SILCS) is a single-size silicone contoured diaphragm which was launched in six European countries in late 2013 including the UK and Germany. It is designed to fit approximately 80% of women. As with other diaphragms it is used with spermicidal gel. It does not require fitting by a health professional however the FSRH recommends assessing women to ensure that the diaphragm fits correctly. **Caps** are smaller than diaphragms and sit directly over the cervix, held in place by suction. The only cervical cap currently available in the UK and USA is the Femcap (Figure 5.3), a silicone device available in three sizes (22 mm, 26 mm and 30 mm). **Sponges:** Contraceptive vaginal sponges are no longer available in the UK. The Today sponge is a polyurethane device impregnated with N-9 available in the USA.

Guidance for users A vaginal examination should be performed by a competent health professional to ensure that the correct size of device is chosen as it must cover the cervix. A further assessment should be made following pregnancy or if a user's weight changes by more than 3 kg. The following advice should be given:

- User should read the manufacturer's instructions
- Spermicide should be applied to the device; two strips to upper side of diaphragm or fill one-third of the cap
- After insertion check the cervix is covered (if not remove and attempt reinsertion)
- Caps and diaphragms can be inserted at any time prior to sex however more spermicide will need to be applied (as a pessary or as cream using an applicator) if sex is to take place and >3 hours has lapsed since the device was inserted or if sex is repeated while method is in place
- The device must be left in situ for a minimum of 6 hours after sex and no longer than the manufacturer recommends. Latex devices can usually be left in situ for a maximum of 30 hours and non-latex devices can be left for up to 48 hours
- After removal wash device in warm water with mild unperfumed soap and allow to air dry
- Check device regularly for signs of damage or perishing

STI prevention: There is little evidence that diaphragms or caps provide protection against transmission of STI's or HIV.

Barrier method failure

Emergency contraception should be considered if a barrier method fails (e.g. condom breakage), or is used incorrectly (see Emergency contraception Chapter 7). STI testing and PEPSE (post-exposure prophylaxis) should also be discussed (see HIV PEPSE).

6 Fertility awareness methods

Figure 6.1 Rhythm method calculation example

Kasey has collected information from her last 6 menstrual cycles

Her longest cycle was 36 days and her shortest cycle was 30 days

She uses the following calculation to predict her fertile days:

First fertile day =
shortest cycle minus 20 (30–20)

Last fertile day =
longest cycle minus 10 (36–10)

Her fertile window begins on day 10 and ends on day 26

During this time she must abstain from sex or use an additional method

---

Figure 6.2 Temperature recording chart

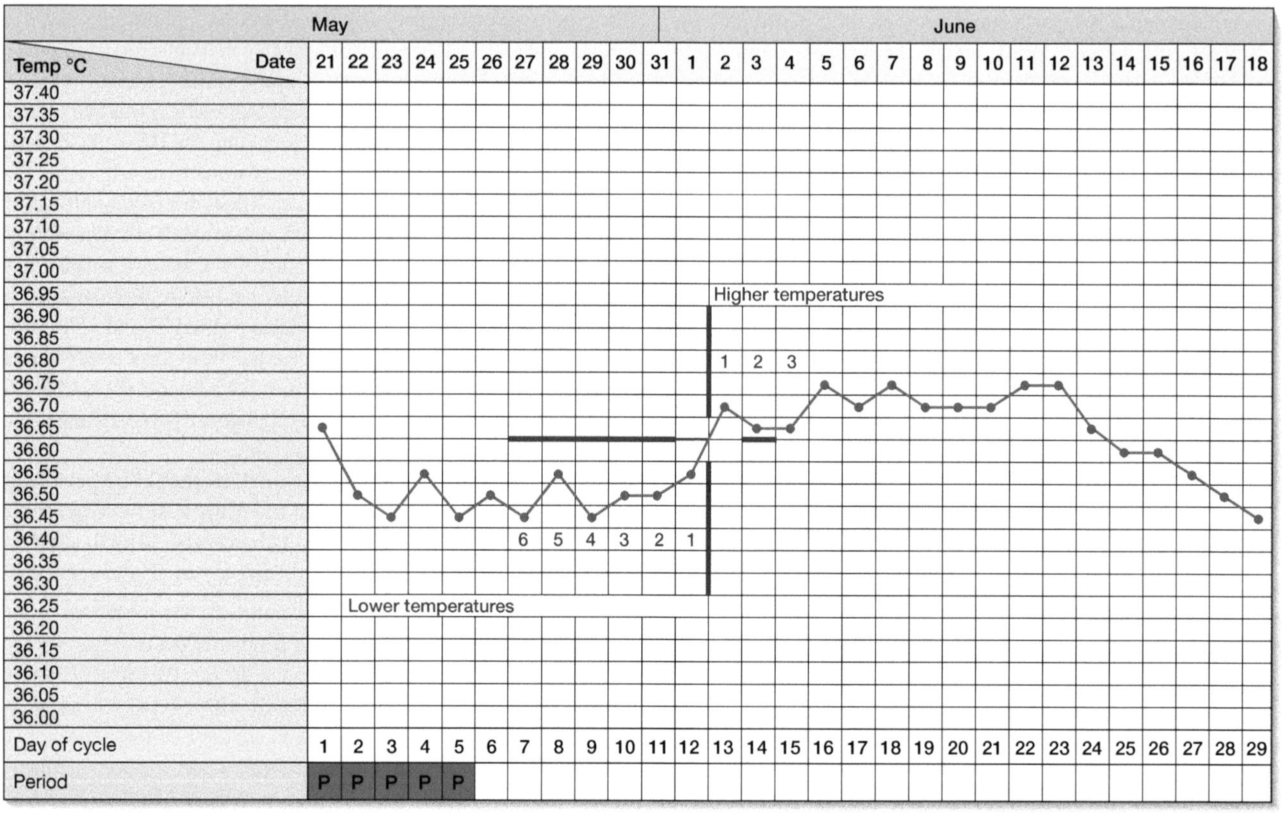

Temp °C / Date	May 21	22	23	24	25	26	27	28	29	30	31	June 1	2	3	4	5	6	7	8	9	10	11	12	13	14	15	16	17	18
37.40																													

Higher temperatures (1 2 3 marked above 36.80 from June 2)

Lower temperatures (countdown 6 5 4 3 2 1 marked near 36.40 on dates 27–31 / June 1)

Day of cycle	1	2	3	4	5	6	7	8	9	10	11	12	13	14	15	16	17	18	19	20	21	22	23	24	25	26	27	28	29
Period	P	P	P	P	P																								

Box 6.1 Fertility awareness methods

Accept Unrestricted use of FAMs

Caution Special counselling may be needed to ensure correct use in these circumstances e.g. use in the first 2 years post-menarche or the peri-menopause

Delay Use of FAM should be delayed until the condition changes or is evaluated e.g. irregular vaginal bleeding or abnormal vaginal discharge

Box 6.2 LAM criteria

Woman must be:
- Less than 6 months postpartum
- Amenorrhoeic
- Exclusively or almost exclusively breastfeeding

Sexual and Reproductive Health at a Glance, First Edition. Catriona Melville. © 2015 by John Wiley & Sons, Ltd. Published 2015 by John Wiley & Sons, Ltd.
Companion website: www.ataglanceseries.com/sexualhealth

Background

Fertility awareness methods (FAMs) or natural family planning (NFP) rely on identifying markers of a woman's fertile period in order to abstain from penetrative sex during the most fertile time. There are three main indicators employed by women using NFP: (1) rhythm method (calendar); (2) temperature method; (3) cervical mucus method

Some methods rely on using only one of the fertility markers whereas others combine two or more. The fertile period is determined by the timing of ovulation. The ovum can survive for up to 24 hours after release from the ovary but is probably only able to be fertilized in the first 12 hours. Average sperm survival is 5 days in the upper reproductive tract; however, sperm can rarely survive for up to 7 days and therefore the fertile period is 8–9 days at most and probably less than this in the majority of women. The reproductive cycle is controlled by the pituitary hormones FSH and LH, which consequently control the release of the ovarian hormones (see Fundamentals Figures 1.2 and 1.3). It is the cyclical changes in the levels of estrogen and progesterone that produce the signs and symptoms of the reproductive cycle which are used to predict the fertile period when using FAMs.

Efficacy is influenced by the age of the women, how often she has sex and the level of adherence with the method. With perfect use, FAMs using a combination of fertility indicators can be up to 99% effective whereas the failure rate of the rhythm method alone is estimated at approximately 20% (range 5–47%). FAMs are most successful when the technique has been taught by trained educators.

Advantages: FAMs have no side effects and are safe and acceptable to all faiths and cultures. They may be chosen by women wishing to avoid artificial contraceptive methods for health concerns or moral reasons.

Disadvantages: It can take several months to become skilled at monitoring the fertility indicators (e.g. 3–6 months) and to collect enough data to start relying on the method. Users must keep daily records which can be difficult to sustain if changes to circumstances occur, e.g. holidays, periods of illness. The period of abstinence can be long in some couples although condoms or another barrier method can be used during these days if acceptable. The method offers no STI protection.

Eligibility: UKMEC categorizes the use of FAMs as 'accept', 'caution' or 'delay' (Box 6.1).

Fertility prediction: FAMs can also be employed to achieve rather than prevent a pregnancy by identifying the fertile period and having sex during the days in which conception is most likely to be achieved.

Rhythm method

Sometimes known as the calendar method of fertility awareness, this is rarely used alone in the UK since by itself it is the least reliable of FAMs. Menstrual cycle length is recorded for a minimum of 6 cycles (12 is preferable) and the likely fertile days are predicted using the survival times of the ovum and sperm. Calculations are based on the longest and shortest recorded menstrual cycles. The period of sexual abstinence is often long using this method alone as in the example in Figure 6.1. The information collected is often used in conjunction with one of the other fertility awareness methods.

Temperature method

Progesterone, the hormone dominant in the post-ovulatory (luteal) phase of the menstrual cycle, has thermogenic properties. Progesterone levels rise during this phase and peak approximately 7 days after ovulation. The rise in progesterone levels causes an increase in basal body temperature (BBT) of 0.2–0.4°C. The BBT is charted daily throughout the menstrual cycle. The recording of three consecutive high temperatures (>0.2°C higher than the six preceding temperatures) indicates the end of the fertile phase (Figure 6.2). Temperatures must be measured before getting out of bed in the morning or after at least 3 hours rest (BBT or waking temperature) and before having anything to eat or drink. Temperature can be measured orally, vaginally or rectally using a special fertility thermometer (mercury or digital), which has widely space markings at 0.1°C. This method may be inaccurate if a febrile illness or infection occurs or if any drugs with antipyretic properties are taken, e.g. paracetamol, aspirin.

Cervical mucus method

This method is sometimes known as the Billings or ovulation method and relies on recognition of cyclical changes in cervical secretions. The colour, amount and texture of cervical mucus is observed and documented daily. Following menses there may be several dry days with no visible mucus at the vulva. In the subsequent days under the influence of increasing estrogen levels, the mucus will change from being scanty and white or cream to copious, clear watery and slippery (like raw egg white). This is the 'fertile mucus' and the last day on which this occurs is termed the 'peak mucus day'. Intercourse is allowed on dry days and resumed on the fourth day after the peak mucus. This method may be used alone or combined with other FAMs. Some users will also use cervical palpation which relies on self-examination for cyclical changes to the consistency and position of the cervix.

Electronic monitoring

Computerized devices measure changes in temperature, urine or saliva. Many of the available monitors are designed to identify the fertile time to aid conception rather than for contraception. Electronic urine testing devices interpret fertile periods based on measurements of LH and estrogen. These devices can be costly to the user. The Marquette method employs a fertility monitor in combination with physiological fertility methods.

Lactation amenorrhoea method (LAM)

Breastfeeding suppresses ovulation by disrupting the frequency and amplitude of gonadotrophin pulses. As the duration and frequency of breastfeeding declines (e.g. over time or with the introduction of supplementary feeds), ovarian activity resumes and ovulation occurs.

In order to use LAM as a contraceptive method, the three criteria in Box 6.2 must be fulfilled. **Efficacy:** LAM is 98% effective if used as recommended. If the frequency of breastfeeding declines (e.g. stopping night feeds), menstruation returns or when the women is over 6 months postpartum, the risk of pregnancy when using LAM is increased.

Resources

http://www.fertilityuk.org/
http://nfp.marquette.edu/
Pyper CMM, Knight J, Fertility awareness methods of family planning: the physiological background, methodology and effectiveness of fertility awareness methods. *Journal of Family Planning and Reproductive Health Care* 2001;27:103–110.

7 Emergency contraception

Figure 7.1 Options for emergency contraception

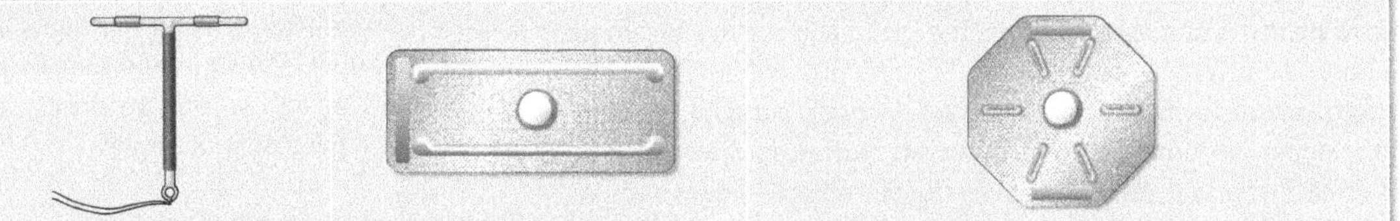

	Cu-IUD	Levonorgestrel (LNG)	Ulipristal acetate (UPA)
Indications	Insert up to 5 days (120 hours) after the first UPSI in the cycle or up to 5 days after the earliest predicted date of ovulation	Licensed use up to 72 hours after UPSI or contraceptive failure 72 – 120 hours after UPSI out with licence	Licensed use up to 120 hours after UPSI or contraceptive failure (the only licensed option for oral EC after 72 hours)
Dose/device	Device should contain 380 mm² of copper and ideally have banded arms	1.5 mg orally stat*	30 mg orally stat*
Efficacy	Pregnancy rate < 1% Most effective method	Pregnancy rate 2.2%† (0 – 120 hours since UPSI) Efficacy after 96 hours is uncertain	Pregnancy rate 1.3%† (0 – 120 hours since UPSI) No decline in efficacy over the 120-hour period
Mode of action	Primary mode is inhibition of fertilization. Anti-implantation effect if fertilisation has already occurred	Delays ovulation by 5 – 7 days if given before the LH surge by which time any sperm in the upper reproductive tract will be non-viable (ineffective after onset of LH surge)	Inhibition or delay of ovulation Effective after the LH surge has started (but before the peak) Delays follicular rupture until up to 5 days later
Drug interactions	N/A	Liver enzyme-inducing drugs may reduce the efficacy of LNG and this effect persists for 28 days afterwards. A Cu-IUD should be offered to all women using these drugs. If a Cu-IUD is unsuitable or unacceptable then a double single dose (3 mg) of LNG is recommended (out with product licence)	Drugs which increase the gastric pH (e.g. proton pump inhibitors, antacids) may result in a decrease in the efficacy of UPA therefore concomitant use is not advised. Liver enzyme-inducing drugs may reduce plasma concentrations of UPA, and therefore an alternative method should be sought for women taking these drugs and for 28 days thereafter. UPA is a PRM and therefore may interfere with progestogen-containing contraceptives. Extra precautions are recommended for 7 days in addition to the number of days required for starting hormonal contraception (Table 7.1)
Contraindications	Very few and the same as for routine insertion (see chapter 4 Intrauterine Contraception)	None	Hypersensitivity to UPA or other components Pregnancy Severe asthma uncontrolled by oral glucocorticoids Use with caution in: hepatic dysfunction, hereditary problems of galactose intolerance, the Lapp lactase deficiency or glucose-galactose malabsorption (because the product contains lactose monohydrate)
Side effects	Pain during insertion	Nausea (< 20% users), headache and altered bleeding patterns (menstruation typically 1.2 days earlier than expected)	Nausea, headache and altered bleeding patterns (menstruation typically 2 days later than expected and delayed by more than 7 days in 20% of women)
Use in breastfeeding women	No restrictions	No restrictions	Detected in breast milk for up to 5 days after ingestion; advised to express and discard breast milk for 7 days after treatment with UPA

* Current recommendations support the use of this dose in obese women
† Reference: Glasier AF, Cameron ST, Logan SJS, Casale W, Van Horn J, Sogar L, et al. Ulipristal acetate versus levonorgestrel for emergency contraception: a randomised non-inferiority trial and meta-analysis. *Lancet* 2010; 375: 555–562

Table 7.1 Requirements for additional precautions after oral EC (condoms or abstinence)

	Ongoing contraceptive method		
Oral EC method	COC	POP	Qlaira
LNG	7 days	2 days	9 days
UPA	14 days	9 days	16 days

N.B. The copper IUD can be used as an ongoing method or removed with next menses and is effective immediately

Figure 7.2 Timing of Cu-IUD insertion

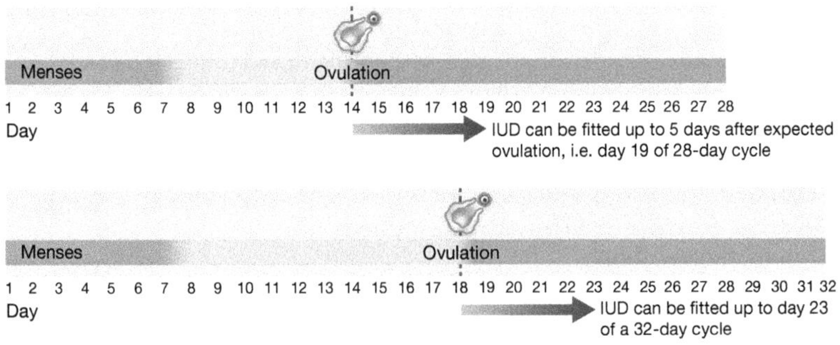

Menses   Ovulation

1 2 3 4 5 6 7 8 9 10 11 12 13 14 15 16 17 18 19 20 21 22 23 24 25 26 27 28
Day → IUD can be fitted up to 5 days after expected ovulation, i.e. day 19 of 28-day cycle

Menses   Ovulation

1 2 3 4 5 6 7 8 9 10 11 12 13 14 15 16 17 18 19 20 21 22 23 24 25 26 27 28 29 30 31 32
Day → IUD can be fitted up to day 23 of a 32-day cycle

The luteal phase (ovulation to menstruation) of the menstrual cycle is relatively constant at 14 days; however, the follicular phase is more variable. In a regular 28-day cycle the Cu-IUD can be inserted safely up to day 19

Sexual and Reproductive Health at a Glance, First Edition. Catriona Melville. © 2015 by John Wiley & Sons, Ltd. Published 2015 by John Wiley & Sons, Ltd.
Companion website: www.ataglanceseries.com/sexualhealth

Background

Emergency contraception (EC) is indicated when a woman's routine contraception has failed (e.g. missed or late method use, concurrent use of enzyme-inducing drugs, severe diarrhoea), or when unprotected sexual intercourse (UPSI) has occurred. There are currently three options for emergency contraception (Figure 7.1): Cu-IUD, Levonorgestrel (LNG) and Ulipristal acetate (UPA).

- The requirement for emergency contraception and the choice will depend on factors such as likely pregnancy risk, contraindications and patient preference
- Pregnancy risk: Sperm can survive for 5 days in the upper reproductive tract (an absolute maximum of 7 days) and the unfertilized ovum can survive for around 24 hours. The highest risk of pregnancy from a single act of UPSI is therefore in the 24 hours prior to ovulation or the day of ovulation itself. The risk of pregnancy is lowest at the start and end of the menstrual cycle, e.g. days 1–9 and days 18–28 of a 28-day cycle
- If there has been a risk of pregnancy there may also be a risk of STI exposure, either from this or preceding episodes of UPSI, so an STI risk assessment should be undertaken and consideration given to screening for STIs
- A pregnancy test may be indicated particularly if there has been a risk earlier in the cycle. Pregnancy cannot be reliably excluded until 3 weeks after an episode of UPSI

Cu-IUD

- The Cu-IUD is the most effective method of emergency contraception and should be offered to all eligible women
- Copper is toxic to both the sperm and ovum and therefore prevents fertilization. It is not an abortifacient
- When calculating the earliest date of ovulation for Cu-IUD insertion, measurement should be based on the shortest cycle length (Figure 7.2)
- Age, nulliparity, risk of STIs and previous ectopic pregnancy are NOT contraindications to use
- No additional precautions are required following Cu-IUD use for EC as it is immediately effective
- The LNG-IUS is not effective for emergency contraception and should not be used

Levonorgestrel

- Levonorgestrel for use as progestogen only emergency contraception (POEC) is widely licensed worldwide
- It is marketed as Levonelle® (UK, Australia, New Zealand), Plan B One-Step® (USA, Canada) and Norlevo® (Asia, Africa, Western Europe)
- In the UK it is available for purchase at pharmacies without a prescription as Levonelle One Step®

Ulipristal acetate

- Known as ellaOne® in Europe and Ella® in the USA, this oral method of EC was launched in 2009
- UPA is a selective progesterone receptor modulator (SPRM). If a woman chooses to continue with a pregnancy after failed UPA this should be reported to the manufacturer to enable them to monitor outcomes of exposure in pregnancy

Which option to choose?

- The Cu-IUD is the most effective method of emergency contraception and should be offered to all eligible women
- UPA is more expensive than LNG; however, for those women at high risk of conception e.g. mid-cycle UPSI or if >72–120 hours since UPSI, it may be recommended

Vomiting after oral emergency contraception

- LNG: if vomiting occurs within 2 hours of treatment then a repeat dose is indicated
- UPA: if vomiting occurs within 3 hours of treatment a repeat dose is indicated

Repeat use of oral EC in a cycle

- If LNG fails to prevent a pregnancy there is no evidence of adverse pregnancy outcomes or congenital malformations. LNG does not induce an abortion. If further episodes of UPSI occur in the same cycle, then a repeat dose of LNG can be given (out with product licence). Further EC treatment is not required within 12 hours of a dose of LNG
- UPA should not be given more than once in a cycle as there is limited data about its safety in pregnancy. It should not be given concomitantly with LNG but LNG can be given after UPA for another risk following UPSI in the same cycle

Follow-up

- Women should be advised to attend for a pregnancy test if menses do not occur within 3 weeks of EC
- After Cu-IUD insertion, follow-up is recommended after the first menses or 3 weeks. If removal is requested this can be undertaken after pregnancy has been excluded, provided there has been no UPSI in the 7 days prior to removal
- Further STI testing may be indicated at follow-up
- Ongoing contraception should be discussed

Meeting ongoing contraceptive needs

- LNG and UPA do not provide contraceptive cover for any further episodes of UPSI in that cycle
- The Cu-IUD can be continued for ongoing contraception
- Women may either wait until pregnancy is excluded to start a hormonal method of contraception or consider 'quick starting' or resuming their existing method

'Quick starting' contraception

- Refers to starting contraception at the time of request rather than delaying it until the next menstrual cycle. This is outside the product licence for hormonal methods, the LNG-IUS and some Cu-IUDs, but is recommended in National guidelines
- After EC, the COC, POP or PO implant can be started immediately if this is acceptable to the woman and she understands the importance of follow-up to exclude pregnancy (i.e. advised to have a pregnancy test in ≥3 weeks)
- If pregnancy is diagnosed DMPA cannot be removed or stopped; therefore, it should only be quick started if other methods are not suitable or acceptable
- An LNG-IUS should never be inserted until pregnancy is excluded and a Cu-IUD should only be inserted if the requirements for its use as EC are met
- If pregnancy is diagnosed after quick starting and the women wishes to continue with the pregnancy then the method should be stopped
- If continuing or quick starting a hormonal contraceptive method, additional precautions are required (Table 7.1)
- Advanced supply of oral EC has not been shown to reduce pregnancy rates; however, it can be considered on individual basis

8 Male and female sterilization

Box 8.1 Sterilization counselling

- Ideally conduct with both men and women together
- Include information on sterilisation procedures including anaesthesia
- Include information on other contraceptive methods including LARC
- Highlight the permanence of sterilisation
  (reversal not usually available on the NHS)
- Explore the myths associated with sterilization, e.g. vasectomy does not cause impotence, loss of desire, affect ejaculation or prevent orgasm
- Include information regarding risks, complications and failure rates
- Advise that vasectomy is safer, quicker and associated with less morbidity than laparotomy or laparoscopic sterilisation
- Explain the requirement for confirmatory tests for vasectomy (PVSA) and hysteroscopic sterilization (and the importance of continuing contraception until such tests are completed)
- Highlight and explore known factors associated with regret (Box 8.2)
- Provide information verbally and in writing and document in the patient records

Table 8.1 UKMEC for sterilization

Eligibility category	
Accept	No medical reason that sterilisation cannot be undertaken in a person with this condition
Caution	Undertake the procedure in a routine setting but extra precautions or counselling may be required, e.g. individuals < 30 years of age
Delay	Delay procedure until the condition is evaluated (and/or changes). Alternative method of contraception should be offered meantime, e.g. uncontrolled hypertension
Special	Experienced surgeon/staff and equipment for general anaesthesia, e.g. coagulation disorder

For further information consult http://www.fsrh.org/pdfs/UKMEC2009.pdf

Figure 8.3 Post-vasectomy semen analysis: PVSA

- Approximately 80% of men will be azoospermic by 12 weeks post-vasectomy or after 20 ejaculations
- PVSA should be undertaken no earlier than 12 weeks postoperatively
- A routine second sample is not required if the first test demonstrates azoospermia
- 'Special clearance' to stop contraception can be given if < 100 000 non-motile sperm/ml are found in a fresh specimen examined at least 3 months post-vasectomy

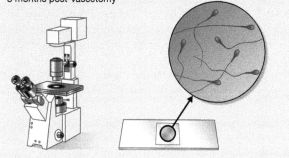

Box 8.2 Factors associated with regret

- Young age (especially under 30)
- Few or no children
- Within a year of birth, miscarriage or induced abortion
- Recent loss of a child
- Relationship crisis or not in mutually faithful relationship
- Not in a relationship
- Coercion by a partner or a health professional
- Lack of information about procedure
- Partner opposed to procedure

Figure 8.1 Anatomy pre- and post-vasectomy

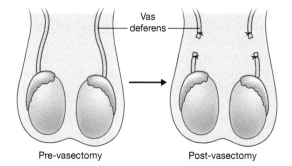

Vas deferens

Pre-vasectomy   Post-vasectomy

Figure 8.2 NSV

No scalpel fixation ring clamp
(secures vas through scrotal skin)

No scalpel dissecting forceps
(punctures scrotum)

Sexual and Reproductive Health at a Glance, First Edition. Catriona Melville. © 2015 by John Wiley & Sons, Ltd. Published 2015 by John Wiley & Sons, Ltd.
Companion website: www.ataglanceseries.com/sexualhealth

Background

Worldwide, sterilization is the most common form of contraception in use. One-fifth of married women use female sterilization as their contraceptive method, resulting in 225 million users of this method. By contrast, vasectomy is less popular (and arguably underused) in most countries, with approximately 33 million users worldwide in 2007. In the United Kingdom, the popularity of female sterilization has declined significantly over the past decade. This is postulated to be due to the increased uptake of the extremely reliable long-acting reversible contraceptive (LARC) methods. The total number of vasectomies performed in the UK has also shown a decline over the past decade (2000–2010).

Counselling for male and female sterilization (Boxes 8.1, 8.2)

Ideally counselling for sterilization should take place in a setting where all alternative methods of contraception can be discussed and offered. Counselling should be adequate to ensure valid consent is obtained for the procedure. A medical history should be taken to confirm suitability for the procedure and anaesthetic. In women this should include a menstrual and gynaecological history. History and examination should determine eligibility for the procedure (Table 8.1).

Vasectomy

What is it?

Vasectomy or male sterilization is a permanent method of contraception, whereby the vas deferens are divided or occluded to prevent the passage of sperm from the epididymis (Figure 8.1).

Procedure techniques

Vasectomy can usually be performed under local anaesthesia as a day case or outpatient. The scrotum is opened either by a single midline incision, or by bilateral incisions (one on each side of the scrotum). The exposed fascial sheath is then opened longitudinally and the vas divided. A portion of vas is removed, and the distal and proximal ends of the vas are occluded by a variety of methods. Traditionally the vas is ligated with sutures; however, other methods of vasal occlusion including cautery of the lumen with unipolar diathermy may be used. The fascial sheath can be interposed between the cut ends of the vas. This is termed fascial interposition (FI). This technique appears to reduce vasectomy failure. Randomized trial evidence comparing the efficacy of different techniques is lacking; however, a Cochrane review has suggested that occluding the lumen with cautery, combined with FI is the most effective technique. Irrigation of the vas lumen does not reduce failure rates, and the use of clips to occlude the vas is no longer recommended due to an unacceptably high failure rate. The excised portions of vas do not routinely need to be sent for histological analysis.

A minimally invasive vasectomy (MIV) technique known as the no-scalpel vasectomy (NSV) was developed in China in the 1970s and is associated with lower rates of haematoma and infection (Figure 8.2). A small clamp is used to hold the vas through the scrotal skin and then a sharp tipped dissecting forceps is used to puncture the scrotum (rather than incise it). MIV techniques to isolate the vas deferens are regarded as the methods of choice, but many surgeons world-wide still employ the traditional scalpel method.

Advantages

Vasectomy is a safe and effective method of permanent contraception, which can usually be performed without the need for a general anaesthetic.

Disadvantages

Unlike other methods of contraception, vasectomy requires a surgical procedure with its associated risk of complications. It is not immediately effective, and it is not easily reversed.

Complications

All men will experience some discomfort, bruising and swelling in the first few postoperative days. Recognized complications are:

* scrotal haematoma: affects 1–2% of men but can usually be managed with scrotal support and analgesia. Occasionally it necessitates admission to hospital for drainage
* wound infection occurs in up to 1% of men
* epididymitis: blockage of the epididymis leads to pressure and pain in less than 6% of men. This usually settles on its own
* sperm granuloma: small lumps caused by a local inflammatory response can occur due to sperm leakage from the cut ends of the vas (risk 2 in 100). This usually settles but may require surgical excision
* Chronic testicular or scrotal pain (post-vasectomy syndrome): The quoted incidence ranges from 12–52%; however, these figures are based mainly on questionnaire studies so are likely to be an overestimate. Pain may result from scar tissue forming around the fine nerve fibres or be due to granuloma formation of the epididymis and vas deferens. The pain is not usually severe but can be long lasting

Stopping contraception: PVSA

Before relying on vasectomy for contraception, men must complete post vasectomy semen analysis (PVSA). The purpose of this is to confirm success of the procedure or identify early failure. There is no consensus regarding the recommended number and timing of PVSA samples and it is usually determined locally. Traditionally men submitted two samples of sperm, a month apart. If both showed complete absence of sperm then 'clearance' was given and the vasectomy could be relied on for contraception. Recent guidance supports the demonstration of a single azoospermia specimen to confirm clearance. In a small number of men (1.4–2.5%), non-motile sperm persist after vasectomy. 'Special clearance' can be given in some circumstances (Fig 8.3). In countries where PVSA is unavailable, a recommended number of ejaculations are suggested to clear sperm before other contraceptive use can be ceased.

Efficacy

The lifetime failure rate of vasectomy is 1 in 2000 after clearance is given. Early or operative failure can occur due to technical failure (e.g. wrong structure occluded) or early recanalization of the vas. It is identified by failure to achieve azoospermia in the PVSA specimens. The early failure rate should be less than 1%. Late failures occur due to recanalization of the vas deferens and may take place many years after the procedure. Late failures are defined as the presence of sperm in ejaculates after confirmation of sterility (azoospermia or special clearance at PVSA).

Figure 8.4 Female sterilization: tubal occlusion

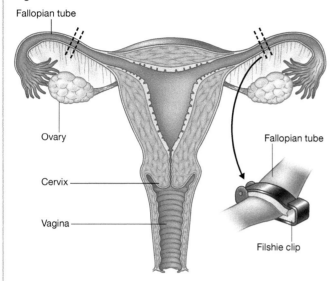

Fallopian tube

Ovary

Cervix

Vagina

Fallopian tube

Filshie clip

Figure 8.5 Pomeroy technique

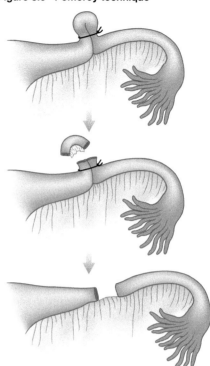

Figure 8.6 Hysteroscopic sterilization with Essure®

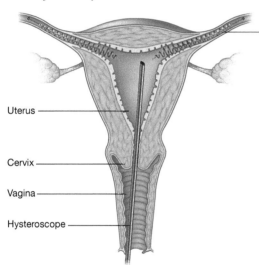

Essure micro-insert in Fallopian tube

Uterus

Cervix

Vagina

Hysteroscope

Box 8.3 Complications of laparoscopic sterilization

- Damage to bowel or major blood vessels (0.4/1000 and 0.2/1000 respectively)
- Conversion to laparotomy
- Complications of anaesthesia
- Risk of death associated with the procedure is 1 in 12 000

N.B. Complications are more common in obese patients and those who have had previous abdominal surgery or pelvic infection

Box 8.4 Female sterilization: key points

- Laparoscopic sterilization under general anaesthetic using Filshie clips is the most common method used in the UK
- Transcervical (hysteroscopic) sterilization is emerging as a safe and efficacious alternative to the abdominal approach
- In developing countries, mini-laparotomy is common and chemical methods such as quinacrine pellets are used

Reversal of vasectomy

During preoperative counselling men should be made aware that vasectomy is intended to be permanent. A common reason for reversal request is when a new relationship is started. There is wide variation in the quoted success rates of vasectomy reversal (between 50–80%). The successful reversal and subsequent pregnancy rates decrease with time since vasectomy, with much lower success rates after 10 years. This decline in success over time may reflect the presence of antisperm antibodies; however, their significance is unclear. In the UK, reversal of vasectomy is rarely available within the NHS and there are therefore cost implications for the individual.

Vasectomy and disease

There is no evidence that vasectomy increases the risk of heart disease or testicular cancer. There is an association in some reports of an increased risk of being diagnosed with prostate cancer; however, it is currently considered that this is likely to be a non-causative association.

Female sterilization

What is it?

The fallopian tubes are occluded (by a variety of approaches and techniques) impeding sperm transport to the ampulla of the tube, where fertilization of the ovum occurs (Figure 8.4).

Techniques

Abdominal approach

Worldwide, this is the most commonly used method of accessing the fallopian tubes in order to occlude them. Laparoscopic female sterilization is most commonly used in the UK and USA; however, in the developing world, due to lack of equipment, facilities and expertise in laparoscopic surgery, most sterilization procedures are carried out using a mini-laparotomy. Occlusion can be achieved using:

- **Mechanical methods**: A clip or ring is applied to each tube. A titanium clip, the Filshie clip, is most often used in the UK and is applied as right angles to the isthmic portion of the tube, 1–2 cm from the cornu and completely encasing the tube
- **Surgical methods**: absorbable sutures are used to tie the tube and a portion is removed. One such technique is the modified Pomeroy or Parkland technique (Figure 8.5). Although tying and ligating the tubes is not used first line in most developed countries, it appears to have a place in post-partum sterilization where it may have a lower failure rate than the application of mechanical methods. The evidence is however conflicting
- **Bipolar diathermy**: this should not be used as a primary method of tubal occlusion as it is more difficult to reverse and is associated with an increased risk of subsequent ectopic pregnancy

Transcervical approach

- **Hysteroscopic sterilization**: This procedure whereby tubal cannulation and placement of intrafallopian implants is used to occlude the tubes mechanically has been supported by NICE in the UK since 2009. The only licensed product, Essure®, has been approved by the EU and US FDA. Essure® is a flexible micro-insert which induces scar formation thereby occluding the fallopian tubes (Figure 8.6). The inflammatory reaction in the tubes peaks at 3 weeks; however, women are advised to use additional contraception for 3 months post procedure. Tubal occlusion is then confirmed using transvaginal ultrasound scan, X-ray or hysterosalpingogram
- **Chemical occlusion:** Blind insertion of quinacrine hydrochloride pellets into the uterine cavity has been used for many years in developing countries. Quinacrine causes fibrosis of the endothelial lining of the proximal part of the Fallopian tubes. This method is not licensed in the UK. Quinacrine sterilization was banned in India in 1998 due to concerns regarding potential teratogenicity and carcinogenicity although these concerns have not been substantiated and research from countries such as Vietnam and Chile, where the method has been used for many years have demonstrated an acceptable safety profile

Anaesthesia and analgesia

The majority of laparoscopic female sterilizations in the UK are performed as day cases under general anaesthesia. Post-procedure pain, thought to be due to tubal ischaemia can be reduced by topical application of local anaesthetic to the tubes either before or after occlusion. Local anaesthesia (with or without sedation) can be used as an alternative to general anaesthesia.

Hysteroscopic sterilization can be performed with either local anaesthetic, and/or intravenous sedation, or in some cases without the need for anaesthetic at all.

Advantages

- Method independent of sexual intercourse
- High efficacy
- Permanent
- Non-hormonal method

Disadvantages

- Surgical procedure required with the associated risks
- Often requires a general anaesthetic
- Permanent
- Offers no STI protection
- Increased risk of ectopic pregnancy if fails

Complications of laparoscopy – Box 8.3

Efficacy

The lifetime failure rate of tubal occlusion is estimated as 1 in 200. The Filshie clip has a 10-year failure rate of 2–3 per 1000 procedures. It is estimated that Essure® is 99.8% effective in pregnancy prevention at two-year follow-up.

Contraception

A pregnancy test should be performed routinely on the day of surgery however this will not identify a luteal-phase pregnancy therefore women should be advised to use a reliable method of contraception in the month preceding the sterilization and until their next menstrual period.

Key points – Box 8.4

Contraception for specific groups of individuals

9

Figure 9.1 Addressing young people's concerns about contraception

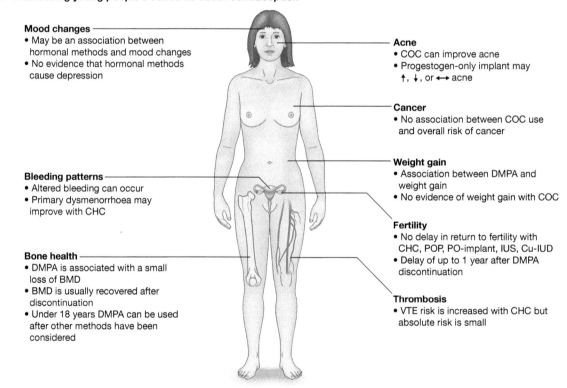

Mood changes
• May be an association between hormonal methods and mood changes
• No evidence that hormonal methods cause depression

Bleeding patterns
• Altered bleeding can occur
• Primary dysmenorrhoea may improve with CHC

Bone health
• DMPA is associated with a small loss of BMD
• BMD is usually recovered after discontinuation
• Under 18 years DMPA can be used after other methods have been considered

Acne
• COC can improve acne
• Progestogen-only implant may ↑, ↓, or ↔ acne

Cancer
• No association between COC use and overall risk of cancer

Weight gain
• Association between DMPA and weight gain
• No evidence of weight gain with COC

Fertility
• No delay in return to fertility with CHC, POP, PO-implant, IUS, Cu-IUD
• Delay of up to 1 year after DMPA discontinuation

Thrombosis
• VTE risk is increased with CHC but absolute risk is small

Table 9.1 Initiation of contraceptive methods in postpartum women: UKMEC

Breastfeeding or non-breastfeeding women (regardless of mode of delivery)

• POP: anytime from delivery UKMEC 1
• *PO-implant*: anytime from delivery UKMEC 1 (although prior to day 21 is out with product licence)
• POEC: not required before day 21
  ≥ 21 days UKMEC 1
• Diaphragms/caps: ≥ 6 weeks UKMEC 1 (attend for assessment and fitting at this time)
• Condoms: anytime from delivery UKMEC 1
• Cu-IUD: 48 hours to 4 weeks UKMEC 3
  ≥ 4 weeks UKMEC 1
• LNG-IUS: 48 hours to 4 weeks UKMEC 3
  ≥ 4 weeks UKMEC 1

Breastfeeding women

• CHC: < 6 weeks UKMEC 4
  ≥ 6 weeks to 6 months UKMEC 3 (partial breastfeeding UKMEC 2)
  > 6 months UKMEC 1
• *PO-injectables*: < 6 weeks UKMEC 2 (postpone first injection until 21 days)
  ≥ 6 weeks UKMEC 1

Non-breastfeeding women

• *CHC*: < 21 days (UKMEC 3)
  ≥ 21 days (UKMEC 1)
• *PO-injectables*: UKMEC 1 at anytime from delivery

Sexual and Reproductive Health at a Glance, First Edition. Catriona Melville. © 2015 by John Wiley & Sons, Ltd. Published 2015 by John Wiley & Sons, Ltd.
Companion website: www.ataglanceseries.com/sexualhealth

Young people

Consent, capacity and confidentiality

In the UK, any young person can give consent to medical treatment (including contraception) as long as they are deemed competent. In law, all people over 16 years of age are presumed to be competent and have the capacity to give consent. Those under 16 years old however must demonstrate their competence to consent by meeting standards set by the Courts.

- In England, Wales, and Northern Ireland the young person must be deemed to have enough understanding and be mature enough to understand fully what is proposed
- In Scotland the young person must be capable of understanding the nature and possible consequences of the treatment

The Fraser Guidelines/criteria (Box 9.1) are used to assess capacity for provision of contraception in under 16s in England, Wales and Northern Ireland. Although often used by HCPs, these guidelines have no standing in Scottish Law. Instead, competency in Scotland is governed by the Age of Legal Capacity (Scotland) Act 1991.

The duty of confidentiality to all patients is irrespective of age. This includes circumstances in which a breach of confidentiality may be justified, e.g. child protection concerns. Young people should be informed of confidentiality policies including situations in which it may need to be breached. Key resources are listed in Box 9.2.

Contraceptive choices

On the basis of age alone in young people, all contraceptive methods are awarded a UKMEC category 1 or 2. This includes the intrauterine methods which should be offered to young people. The benefits of the LARC methods in terms of efficacy and convenience should be emphasized. Young people may have specific concerns regarding side effects and health risks of contraceptive methods (Figure 9.1). Addressing these issues and particularly any misconceptions may improve adherence to a method.

Initiation of contraception should follow the method-specific guidance. Quick-starting contraception can be a useful option in young people. Follow-up should be undertaken at 3 months or at any time if there are questions or concerns. Information should be given about emergency contraception and also STI testing.

Postpartum women

- Non-breastfeeding women: Contraception is required from day 21 as the earliest date of ovulation is Day 28. Menstruation may return by week 6
- Breastfeeding women: LAM can be used alone in fully breastfeeding women until criteria are no longer met or breastfeeding reduces (see Chapter 6)

Effect of contraceptive hormones in breast milk

Contraceptive hormones are excreted into breast milk in very small amounts, raising concerns about potential adverse consequences on infant growth or development and breastfeeding. For this reason some limitations are placed on use of these methods in breastfeeding women. Current evidence however suggests that infant developmental outcomes do not appear to be affected by hormonal contraceptive methods.

Progestogen-only contraception

- Breast milk volume is not affected
- No effect has been shown on infant growth or development

CHC

- Should be avoided for the first 6 weeks post delivery in breastfeeding women as there is a lack of evidence to support the safety of use while establishing breastfeeding (UKMEC 4)
- Not recommended in fully breastfeeding women in the first 6 months postpartum unless other methods unacceptable (UKMEC 3)

Initiation of contraceptive methods

The eligibility criteria given to initiation of different contraceptive methods in the postpartum period are summarized in Table 9.1. CHC should not be initiated within 21 days postpartum due to the increased risk of VTE (UKMEC 3). Non-breastfeeding women can commence these methods from day 21 (UKMEC 1). Different categories may be awarded for breastfeeding women. The SPC for methods may differ from the UKMEC category. Do not insert an intrauterine device or system in the presence of puerperal sepsis (UKMEC 4). Initiation of injectable progestogens in the early postpartum period can be associated with troublesome bleeding in some women.

Other issues in postpartum women

Sexual problems can occur in the postpartum period (e.g. dyspareunia) and women should be given the opportunity to discuss any concerns with a HCP supported by appropriate management. As with any contraceptive discussion, consideration should be given to the need for protection against STIs and/or screening.

Women in the later reproductive years

Contraceptive choices

Although fertility in women declines with age and particularly from the mid-30s, in order to avert unplanned pregnancy, contraception must be continued until after the menopause. As with younger women, the choice of contraceptive methods in older women should not be restricted by age alone. As women age however, it may be more likely that medical co-morbidities exist, e.g. hypertension, which can preclude use of certain methods of contraception.

Figure 9.2 Health concerns and issues related to contraceptive methods in women > 40 years

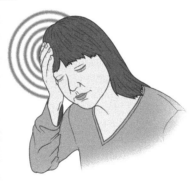

CVS and cerebrovascular disease
CHC
- Use → v. small↑ risk of ischaemic stroke
- Risk↑ further in ♀ who have migraine with aura
- Risk of MI increases in COC users who smoke

POC
- No increased risk of stroke or MI
- DMPA adversely affects lipids so caution advised when ♀ presenting for with risk factors

Dysmenorrhea and bleeding patterns
CHC
- May ↓ menstrual pain and bleeding

POC
- Altered bleeding patterns common
- LNG-IUS helpful in managing HMB

Cu-IUD
- May be associated with heavy or prolonged bleeding, dysmenorrhea and spotting

VTE risk
CHC
- COC use associated with small increase in risk of VTE
- Risk may↓ by ↓ dose of estrogen in COC, e.g. 20 µg instead of 30 µg

POC
- No increased risk of VTE

Symptoms of the menopause
CHC
- May reduce some menopausal symptoms
- An extended regimen may be beneficial for this

POC
- DMPA may reduce vasomotor symptoms

Breast cancer
CHC
- Small increased risk in current users
- Declines to that of non-users < 10 years of cessation

POC
- No link has been demonstrated between PO menthods and breast cancer

Bone health
CHC
- May help maintain BHD if used in menopause

POC
- DMPA associated with small ↓BMD which usually recovers on cessation of method
- Review DMPA users 2-yearly and discontinue method at maximum age of 50 years

Figure 9.3 Determining the menopause using serum FSH measurements (in women > 50 years)

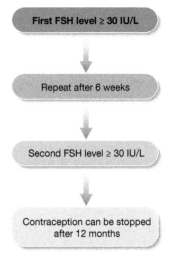

First FSH level ≥ 30 IU/L

↓

Repeat after 6 weeks

↓

Second FSH level ≥ 30 IU/L

↓

Contraception can be stopped after 12 months

Table 9.2 Stopping contraception

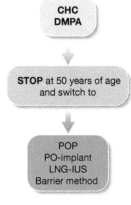

CHC
DMPA

↓

STOP at 50 years of age and switch to

↓

POP
PO-implant
LNG-IUS
Barrier method

Figure 9.4 Features of migraine headache

Symptoms
- Moderate to severe unilateral headache
- Pulsating or throbbing in nature
- Lasts 4 – 72 hours
- May be accompanied by nausea, vomiting, photophobia, phonophobia

Four stages of migraine
1 Prodrome
2 Aura
3 Headache
4 Recovery

Box 9.3 Diagnosing migraine aura

- Visual symptoms occur in 99% of auras
- Aura occurs before the headache
- Aura lasts up to an hour
- Aura resolves before the onset of headache

CHC should not be used in women who have migraine with aura due to the increased risk of ischaemic stroke: UKMEC 4

Table 9.3 UKMEC categories for migraine

	CHC		POP		PO-injectables; PO-implant; LNG-IUS
Migraine without aura*	I 2	C 3	I 1	C 2	2
Migraine with aura*	4		2		2
Past history (≥ 5 years ago) of migraine with aura*	3		2		2

*At any age

I = Initiation of the method in a person with the condition

C = Continuation of the method when a woman develops the new condition while using the method

Use of CHC is awarded a UKMEC 2 in women ≥40years. Injectable progestogens, e.g. DMPA, are awarded a UKMEC 2 in women ≥45 years. All other methods are unrestricted in women over 40 years (UKMEC 1) as long as no coexisting contraindicating factors exist. As with women of any age, the efficacy of LARC methods should be emphasized. In particular, women and their partners should be informed that the failure rates of the vLARC methods are comparable with female sterilization.

Older women's concerns about the significance of some of the health risks and benefits associated with contraception use should be addressed and discussed (Figure 9.2). Furthermore:

- CHC use in women ≥35 years who smoke <15 cigarettes per day is UKMEC 3
- CHC use in women ≥35 years who smoke ≥15 cigarettes per day is UKMEC 4
- CHC use in women with a history of stroke (including TIA), CVS disease or current migraine with aura is not advised (UKMEC 4)

Stopping contraception (Table 9.2)

The average age of the menopause is 51 years. A diagnosis of the menopause is usually made clinically and retrospectively by the cessation of menses (1 year of amenorrhoea). Contraception is required until:

- 2 years after the last menstrual period if <50 years of age
- 1 year after the last menstrual period if ≥50 years of age
- at age 55 years contraception can be stopped (unless regular menses are still occurring)

Use of hormonal contraception can 'mask' the menopause by inducing amenorrhoea or changes in bleeding patterns unrelated to cessation of ovarian function. This can result in difficulty determining when to stop contraception. Although measurement of serum gonadotrophic hormones is not usually helpful in the perimenopause, in these circumstances it can prove useful with the following adjuncts:

- FSH measurement should be restricted to women ≥50 years of age who are using PO-methods
- FSH measurement is not reliable in women using CHC methods
  Measurement and interpretation of serum FSH levels in such a situation are detailed in Figure 9.3.

Stopping intrauterine contraception

LNG-IUS:

- if inserted after the age of 45 years it can be retained for 7 years (off licence) or if amenorrhoeic until the menopause
- if inserted after the age of 45 years and exclusively for management of HMB it can be retained for the duration of symptom control
- device should be removed after the menopause

Cu-IUD:

- Women with a device containing ≥300 mm² copper which was inserted ≥40 years of age can retain the device until the menopause
- Device should be removed after the menopause

HRT and contraception

HRT regimens are not contraceptives and women using HRT who are sexually active and pre-menopausal need to use a separate contraceptive method, e.g. the POP. The LNG-IUS is licensed for endometrial protection and can be used as the progestogen component of HRT in women using estrogen replacement therapy. Such use is licensed for 4 years but is supported off license for up to 5 years. At this time the device must be changed regardless of whether it was inserted over the age of 45 years.

Other issues in women over 40 years

STIs

It is not unusual for men and women in their 40s to embark on new relationships. This is reflected by a rise in STI diagnoses in this age group. Women over 40 years seeking contraceptive advice should have a sexual history taken and be offered STI screening where appropriate. Advice should be given about using condoms to protect against STI acquisition and transmission.

Emergency contraception

Women should be informed of the types of emergency contraception available to them and how to access them should their regular method of contraception fail or not be used.

Contraception and medical conditions

Migraine headache

- *Background* Migraine is an episodic headache disorder affecting up to one third of women during their lifetime. There are two main types of migraine: Migraine without aura (70% of attacks), and migraine with aura (30% of attacks). Features of migraine are summarized in Figure 9.4. Not all four stages occur in every attack or in all patients. *Affect of migraine on contraception* A history of migraine is relevant to users of hormonal contraception because migraine is an independent risk factor for ischaemic stroke, particularly in younger women. The association appears to be confined to sufferers who have migraine with aura. **CHC:** Women with migraine who use the COC have a two- to fourfold increase risk of stroke compared to those who are not using COC. CHC methods are therefore contraindicated in women who suffer from current migraine with aura (Box 9.3 and Table 9.3). **PO-contraceptives:** Use of PO-contraceptive methods are not associated with an increased risk of ischaemic stroke. Similarly non-hormonal methods can be safely used by women with migraine. *Affect of contraception on migraine;* headaches are a common symptom in the first few months after initiation of hormonal contraception. They usually resolve with time. In women taking the COC, migraine may improve or show no change in frequency or severity. Migraine and headache often occur in the pill free interval due to falling estrogen levels. Using an extended regimen and/or shortening the pill free interval can help manage symptoms. Evidence regarding the effect of progestogen-only methods on migraine is lacking; however, anecdotally migraine is more likely to improve in women who achieve amenorrhoea with these methods

Table 9.4 Contraceptive methods and EIADs

Contraceptive efficacy not affected by EIAEDs	Contraceptive efficacy may be reduced by EIAEDs
Intrauterine methods (LNG-IUS, CU-IUD)	CHC methods (pill, patch, vaginal ring)
Progestogen-only injectable (DMPA)	Progestogen-only implant
Barrier methods	POP

Table 9.5 Liver enzyme-inducing AEDs

Drug name (generic)	Potency
Carbamazepine	
Eslicarbazepine acetate	
Oxcarbazepine	Strong inducers
Perampanel	
Phenobarbital	
Phenytoin	
Primidone	
Rufinamide	Less potent inducers
Topiramate	

Table 9.6 Non-liver-enzyme-inducing AEDs

Drug name (generic)
Acetazolamide
Benzodiazepines: clobazem, clonazepam
Ethosuximide
Gabapentin
Lacosamide
Lamotrigine
Levetiracetam
Pregabalin
Sodium valproate
Tiagabine
Vigabatrin
Zonisamide

Figure 9.5 Mechanism of liver enzyme-inducing AEDs' effect on contraceptive efficacy

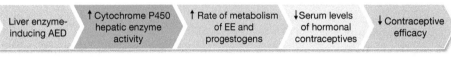

Liver enzyme-inducing AED → ↑ Cytochrome P450 hepatic enzyme activity → ↑ Rate of metabolism of EE and progestogens → ↓ Serum levels of hormonal contraceptives → ↓ Contraceptive efficacy

Figure 9.6 Lamotrigine and CHC

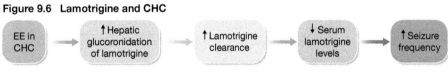

EE in CHC → ↑ Hepatic glucoronidation of lamotrigine → ↑ Lamotrigine clearance → ↓ Serum lamotrigine levels → ↑ Seizure frequency

Table 9.7 IBD and contraception: UKMEC

	Inflammatory bowel disease
CHC	2
POP	2
PO injectable	1
PO implant	1
Cu-IUD	1
LNG-IUS	1
Barrier methods	1

Figure 9.7 Issues related to IBD and contraception

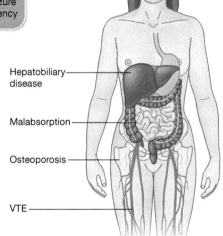

Hepatobiliary disease

Malabsorption

Osteoporosis

VTE

Epilepsy

Background

Epilepsy is a common neurological disorder affecting approximately 1% of the population in the UK. The condition per se does not contraindicate the use of any contraceptive methods, however the drug therapies employed to treat epilepsy may have an effect on contraceptive efficacy (Table 9.4). Additionally, some antiepileptic drugs (AEDs) are affected by hormonal contraceptives which may alter seizure control. The implications of these drug interactions are clinically important as contraceptive failure may arise and furthermore, many anti-epileptic drugs are teratogenic.

Liver enzyme inducing drugs

A number of AEDs induce hepatic cytochrome P450 enzyme activity thus potentially reducing contraceptive efficacy (Figure 9.5 and Table 9.5). Some of these AEDs may be strong enzyme inducers whereas others have a less potent affect (Table 9.5). Intrauterine methods, injectable progestogen-only methods and barrier methods are unaffected by AEDs.

If alternative contraceptives are unsuitable or the AED is being used on a short-term basis only, additional precautions, e.g. a barrier method, must be used for the duration of treatment with the enzyme-inducing AED and for 28 days after cessation.

Lamotrigine (Figure 9.6)

- Lamotrigine is not a liver enzyme-inducing drug (Table 9.6)
- Use of CHC with lamotrigine monotherapy is not recommended (UKMEC 3)
- EE increases the clearance of lamotrigine via hepatic glucoronidation of the drug which results in reduced serum levels of the drug. This can cause an increase in seizure frequency on initiation of a CHC. Conversely serum levels of lamotrigine will increase in the pill free interval or on cessation of the CHC with the potential for drug side effects or toxicity
- Sodium valproate increases serum lamotrigine levels and lessens the effect of CHC
- Lamotrigine may slightly reduce levels of some progestogens, and some progestogens may increase levels of lamotrigine, but the clinical significance of this is not known
- The progestogen-only pill, implant and injectable, and the LNG-IUS and Cu-IUD can be used without restriction (UKMEC 1) with lamotrigine

Emergency contraception

- Efficacy of POEC (LNG) and UPA may be affected by enzyme inducing drugs
- The Cu-IUD should be recommended first-line in women taking an enzyme-inducing drug (or who has stopped one in the last 28 days)
- If only an oral method is acceptable, then 3 mg of LNG (two tablets of Levonelle®) should be given in a single oral dose as soon as possible after UPSI. This is outwith product licence
- There is no supporting evidence for doubling the dose of UPA and its use is not recommended in women who are, or have recently stopped (within 28 days) an enzyme-inducing drug

Bone mineral density (BMD)

Long-term use of some AEDs (carbamazepine, phenytoin, primidone and sodium valproate) is associated with a reduction in BMD in at risk patients. It is unclear whether concomitant use of DMPA compounds this loss, but women using these drugs should be informed of the potential effect on BMD, have a BMD risk assessment and be advised of approaches to maintain bone health.

Inflammatory bowel disease

Background

Inflammatory bowel disease (IBD) consists of two distinct conditions; ulcerative colitis (UC), which affects the large bowel only, and Crohn's disease (CD), which can affect the entire gastrointestinal tract. IBD has a prevalence of approximately 0.1–0.2% and is relevant to SRH as the peak incidence occurs in the reproductive years (ages 20–40 years). IBD is associated with extra-intestinal pathologies such as hepatobiliary disease. Osteoporosis is common in patients with IBD. This may be associated with factors such as corticosteroid use. There is an association between IBD and VTE (Figure 9.7).

Contraceptive issues

Women with IBD should plan to conceive when their disease is well controlled. Some treatments for IBD are teratogenic (e.g. methotrexate) or have unknown effects in pregnancy, emphasizing the requirement for effective contraception during their use (and for a time after cessation). The UKMEC categories for contraception in women with IBD are listed in Table 9.7. Consideration should be given to coexisting pathologies and other risk factors when choosing a method.

- Oral contraception: EE and progestogens are absorbed from the small bowel and therefore small bowel disease and malabsorption may reduce efficacy. Large bowel disease is unlikely to affect efficacy of oral methods
- Progestogen-only injectables and implant, non-oral CHC methods, and intrauterine devices are good alternatives if malabsorption is a concern
- Barrier methods are not reliable enough in women taking teratogenic (or potentially teratogenic) medications. Rectally administered therapies for IBD can in theory spread onto the genital skin and damage barrier methods
- DMPA has possible detrimental effects on BMD and as osteopenia and osteoporosis are more common in women with IBD, consideration should be given to the risks and benefits before using this in those who have the condition
- Laproscopic sterilization in women who have had previous abdominal or pelvic surgery carries twice the complication rate of those with no previous surgery. Hysteroscopic sterilization would be a safe alternative or sterilization at the time of other abdominal surgery
- CHC methods should be stopped at least 4 weeks before major elective surgery to reduce the risks of VTE

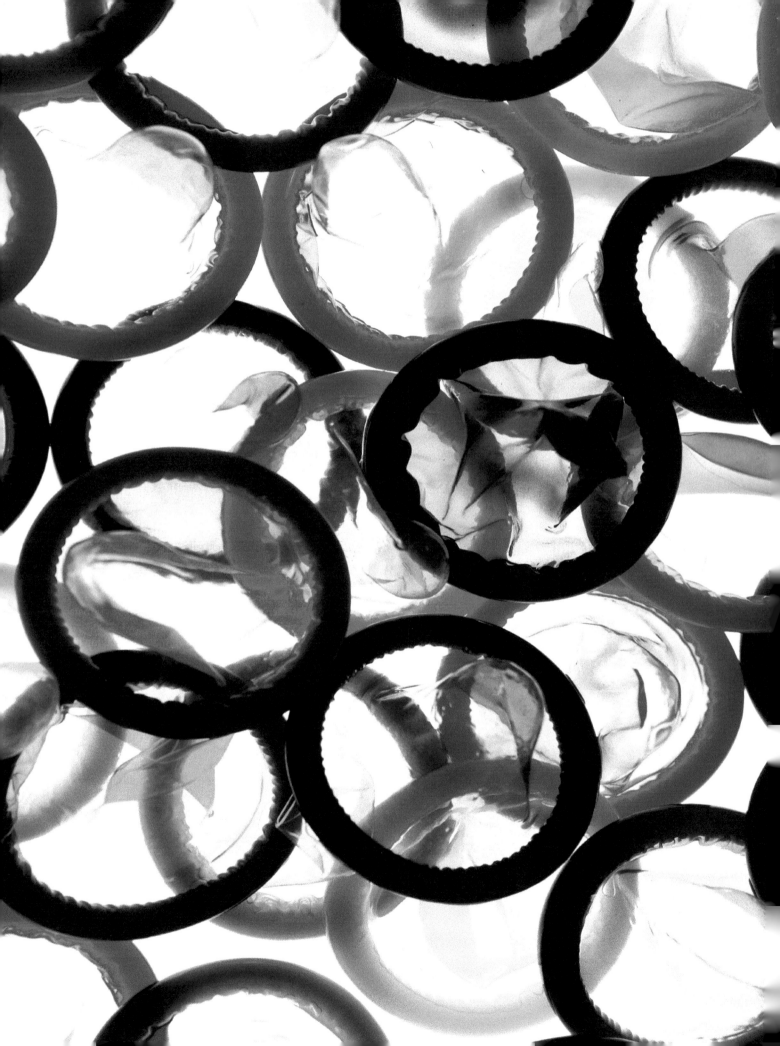

Sexual Health

Part 3

 Don't forget to visit the companion website at www.ataglanceseries.com/sexualhealth where you can test yourself on these topics.

10 Chlamydia trachomatis

Table 10.1 Serovars of *C. trachomatis* which cause human disease

Serovars (serologically variant strains)	Human disease
A, B Ba, C	Hyperendemic trachoma (an endemic eye disease which can lead to blindness)
D-K	Genital tract infections, conjunctivitis
L1, 2, 3	Lymphogranuloma venereum (LGV) Chapter 18

Table 10.2 Chlamydia in pregnancy and the neonate

Pregnancy
• ↑ Risk of premature rupture of the membranes, preterm delivery, low birth weight • ↑ Intrapartum pyrexia • ↑ Postpartum endometritis

Neonates
• Exposed to infection in birth canal during delivery • Approx. 30 – 50% will develop ophthalmia neonatorum (conjunctivitis) • 15% will develop chlamydia pneumonitis

Figure 10.1 Complications of chlamydia infection

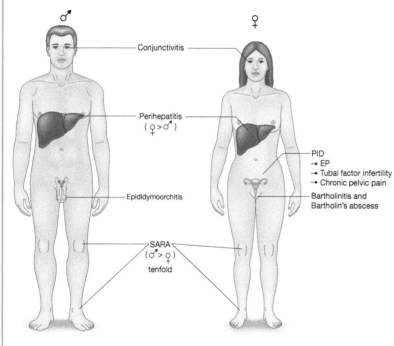

Table 10.3 Treatment of chlamydia

Uncomplicated infections (genital, rectal, pharyngeal)
Azithromycin 1 g orally in a single dose (better compliance but more expensive) *or* Doxycycline 100 mg orally b.d. for 7 days

Alternative regimens
Erythromycin 500 mg orally b.d. 10 – 14 days *or* Ofloxacin 200 mg orally b.d. or 400 mg o.d. for 7 days

Uncomplicated infection in pregnancy*
Azithromycin 1 g orally stat *or* Erythromycin 500 mg orally q.d.s. 7 days *or* Amoxicillin 500 mg orally t.d.s. 7 days

*All three treatments are effective in managing chlamydia in pregnancy; however, compliance may be an issue with erythromycin and amoxicillin due to side effects. Additionally, studies show that penicillins may render the infection latent and it will subsequently reactivate. Azithromycin is not licensed for use in pregnant women, however, its use is supported by WHO and SIGN guidance.

Background

In 2008 the World Health Organization (WHO) estimated there were 105 million new cases of chlamydia worldwide. It is the most frequently reported STI in the USA with 1.4 million cases in 2011. The situation is similar in Europe and the UK where it remains the most commonly diagnosed bacterial STI.

- Aetiology: infection is caused by the obligate intracellular pathogen *Chlamydia trachomatis* which belongs to the genus *Chlamydia*
- Three species of chlamydia cause human disease (Table 10.1)
- Chlamydia predominates in young people with a peak incidence in those under 25 years
- In the UK, 10–15% of sexually active teenagers are infected
- Additional risk factors are a change of partner, non-use or inconsistent use of barrier methods
- Transmission: a single act of UPSI carries a transmission risk of approximately 10% for males and females
- Sites of infections: cervix, urethra, rectum, conjunctiva, pharynx

Symptoms and signs

Females

- Chlamydia is asymptomatic in at least 70% of women
- Symptoms: PCB or IMB, vaginal discharge, dysuria, pelvic pain or deep dyspareunia
- Signs: Cervicitis – a friable cervix which may bleed on contact, ± mucopurulent discharge

Sexual and Reproductive Health at a Glance, First Edition. Catriona Melville. © 2015 by John Wiley & Sons, Ltd. Published 2015 by John Wiley & Sons, Ltd.
Companion website: www.ataglanceseries.com/sexualhealth

Males

- Chlamydia is asymptomatic in 50% of cases
- Symptoms: dysuria or urethral discharge
- Signs: Clear or opaque urethral discharge or urethral meatal oedema and erythema

Rectal infection

- Is usually asymptomatic but can present with anorectal pain and discharge
- Signs: anal discharge, oedema and erythema on proctoscopy

Pharyngeal infection

- typically asymptomatic

Conjunctival infection (adult)

- Symptoms: conjunctival irritation, discharge, photophobia
- Signs: unilateral or bilateral follicular conjunctivitis
- 60–70% will have associated anogenital chlamydia infection

Diagnosis

- A NAAT test is the gold standard diagnostic test for Chlamydia and has replaced enzyme immunoassays (EIAs) and tissue culture
- A variety of commercial NAAT tests are available
- Some assays offer a dual test for *Chlamydia trachomatis* and *Neisseria gonorrhoeae* from a single specimen
- Sample sites: a self-taken lower vaginal swab or an endocervical swab (in women undergoing a speculum) have similar performance and better sensitivity than first-void urine (FVU) in women. In men a FVU is preferable to a urethral swab, which is uncomfortable. Urine must be held for a least an hour before the specimen is taken
- NAATS are not licensed for use with rectal and pharyngeal specimens; however, if indicated, swabs can be taken from these sites and in these circumstances a NAAT is still the test of choice
- Although NAAT tests are highly accurate, no test offers 100% sensitivity and specificity and false-positive results can occur
- Testing interval: individuals should be tested when they first present and if the potential exposure is within the preceding two weeks, they should be re-tested two weeks after exposure

Complications

Both symptomatic and asymptomatic infection can result in complications (Figure 10.1). These include endometritis, bartholinitis and pelvic inflammatory disease (PID), and its sequelae (tubal-factor infertility, ectopic pregnancy and chronic pelvic pain). Ascending infection in men causes epididymo-orchitis. Systemic complications are peri-hepatitis (Fitz-Hugh-Curtis syndrome) and sexually acquired reactive arthritis (SARA). The burden of disease in terms of health care economics is significant.

Complications of chlamydia can also manifest in pregnancy and the neonate (Table 10.2).

Management

Treatment

Treatments for uncomplicated infections are listed in Table 10.3. Regimens for complicated infections, e.g. PID, are given in the relevant chapters.

General

- Advise complete abstinence (no sexual contact even with a condom) until the individual and their partner have been treated, e.g. for 7 days after azithromycin
- Give written information about the infection
- Offer screening for other STIs
- Discuss consistent and correct use of barrier methods

Partner notification

- Approximately two thirds of sexual contacts of the index patient will have chlamydia themselves
- The 'look-back' period for symptomatic infection in men is 4 weeks
- The 'look-back' period for asymptomatic infection in men and infection in women (symptomatic or asymptomatic) is 6 months prior to presentation or until last sexual partner (whichever is longest)
- Contacts should be tested and then treated epidemiologically

Follow-up and test of cure (TOC)

- Follow-up one week after treatment (often by telephone) is useful to confirm adherence to treatment, determine risk of re-infection and check PN
- TOC not routinely recommended as long as therapy has been adhered to and there is no risk of re-infection
- Pregnant women should have a TOC
- TOC should be performed 5 weeks after treatment ends (6 weeks after Azithromycin) to avoid false positive results (as NAATs can identify non-viable organisms)

Chlamydia screening

There is international debate about the optimal strategy for chlamydia screening and testing and a variety of different approaches are therefore used, e.g. targeted, opportunistic or registry-based screening. The natural history of chlamydia infection is not fully understood, however a number of studies demonstrate that about 50% of asymptomatic infections will resolve spontaneously within a year. Also, the complication rates from infection may be much lower than previously believed. PID was thought to occur in up to 40% of untreated women, however the incidence of PID may be as low as 2%. This has obvious implications for the cost-effectiveness of screening programmes.

England introduced the National Chlamydia Screening Programme (NCSP) in 2003. Other countries target testing for certain groups of individuals e.g. sexual health clinic attendees, those undergoing TOP or sexual partners of chlamydia-positive individuals.

New variant chlamydia

A new genetic variant of *C. trachomatis* (nvCT) was discovered in Sweden in 2006; however, some NAAT testing kits available at that time were not capable of detecting this mutation resulting in false-negative results. Isolated cases were found in Scandinavia, France, Ireland and Scotland. Some testing kits have now been modified in order to detect this variant. There is no evidence that this strain of chlamydia causes different disease from the 'normal' strain and infection can be treated with the same antibiotic regimen.

11 Gonorrhoea and non-gonococcal urethritis

Figure 11.1   Gram stain appearance of *N. gonorrhoeae*

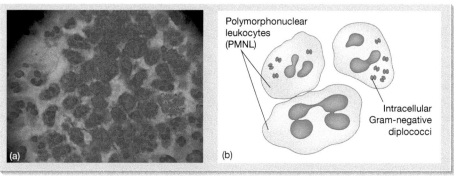

Polymorphonuclear leukocytes (PMNL)

Intracellular Gram-negative diplococci

(a)   (b)

Source: Mark Mason, Senior Specialist Biomedical Scientist, Sandyford, NHS Greater Glasgow & Clyde, Glasgow, UK. Reproduced with permission of Sandyford.

Table 11.1   Treatment of gonorrhoea

Uncomplicated infections (genital, rectal) Ceftriaxone 500 mg i.m. stat*	plus	*Azithromycin 1 g orally stat†
Alternative regimens Cefixime 400 mg orally stat* Should only be used if an i.m. injection is contraindicated or refused	plus	Azithromycin 1 g orally stat†
Spectinomycin 2 g i.m. stat* Use if history of severe hypersensitivity reaction to any cephalosporin/penicillin/other beta-lactam drug		
Pharyngeal infection Ceftriaxone 500 mg i.m. stat *or* Ciprofloxacin 500 mg orally stat (if known to be quinolone-sensitive) *or* Ofloxacin 400 mg orally stat (if known to be quinolone-sensitive)	plus	Azithromycin 1 g orally stat†
Adult gonococcal conjunctivitis (a 3 day systemic course is recommended plus ocular saline irrigation) Ceftriaxone 500 mg i.m. stat daily for 3 days *or* Spectinomycin 2 g i.m. daily for 3 days (if history of severe penicillin allergy)	plus	Azithromycin 1 g orally stat†

For full list of treatment regimens consult current BASHH guidelines Quinolone or tetracycline antimicrobials should not be used in pregnancy or breastfeeding
*These regimens can be used in pregnant women. Azithromycin is not licensed for use in pregnant women; however its use is supported by WHO, BASHH and SIGN guidance.
†Azithromycin is recommended as co-treatment irrespective of the chlamydia result to delay the onset of extensive cephalosporin resistance

Box 11.1   Indications for treatment for gonorrhoea

- Intracellular Gram-negative diplococci identified on microscopy
- Positive NAAT for *N. gonorrhoeae* from any site
- Positive culture for *N. gonorrhoeae* from any site
- Sexual contacts of confirmed cases of gonorrhoea
- Epidemiological treatment may be considered following sexual assault

Table 11.2   Gonorrhoea in pregnancy and the neonate

Pregnancy
- ↑risk of preterm rupture of the membranes, preterm delivery, low birth weight
- ↑intrapartum pyrexia
- ↑postpartum endometritis

Neonates
- Exposed to infection in birth canal during delivery
- Features usually manifest 2 – 5 days after birth
- 30 – 40% will develop gonococcal ophthalmia neonatorum (conjunctivitis)
- Disseminated gonococcal infection can occur especially in preterm infants (sepsis, arthritis, meningitis)

Sexual and Reproductive Health at a Glance, First Edition. Catriona Melville. © 2015 by John Wiley & Sons, Ltd. Published 2015 by John Wiley & Sons, Ltd.
Companion website: www.ataglanceseries.com/sexualhealth

Gonorrhoea

Background

In 2008 the WHO estimated there were 106.1 million new cases of gonorrhoea worldwide. Gonorrhoea diagnosis rates show an upward trend in most European countries. It is the second most common bacterial STI in the UK. New gonorrhoea diagnoses rose by 21% overall in England in 2012 (and by 37% in MSM).

Increasingly gonorrhoea is becoming resistant to antibiotic regimens. The threat of multidrug-resistant gonorrhoea is a global concern.

- Aetiology: infection is caused by the Gram-negative intracellular diplococcus *Neisseria gonorrhoeae*
- The cocci appear in pairs, typically inside polymorphonuclear leucocytes (PMNLs), Figure 11.1
- Risk factors: gonorrhoea is more common in young people, those living in urban areas, MSM and black ethnic minority populations
- Transmission is by direct inoculation of infected secretions from one mucous membrane to another. A single act of UPSI carries a transmission risk of approximately 60–80% for males to females and a 20% risk of infection for females to males
- Primary sites of infection: mucous membranes of the endocervix, urethra, rectum, pharynx and conjunctiva
- Gonorrhoea facilitates the transmission of HIV and may coexist with other STIs especially chlamydia

Symptoms and signs

Females

- 50% endocervical infections will be asymptomatic
- Symptoms: vaginal discharge (up to 50%), dysuria, lower abdominal or pelvic pain, IMB or menorrhagia (rare)
- Signs: examination may be normal or there may be cervicitis with mucopurulent endocervical discharge, easily induced contact bleeding of the cervix, lower abdominal or pelvic tenderness

Males

- 10% urethral infections will be asymptomatic
- Symptoms: urethral discharge (in >80%) and/or dysuria (>50%) commonly within 2–5 days of exposure
- Signs: a purulent or mucopurulent urethral discharge is commonly seen; balanitis, epididymal tenderness or swelling are uncommon

Rectal infection

- In women more often develops by transmucosal spread of infected genital secretions rather than by anal sexual intercourse
- Usually asymptomatic in men and women but can cause anal discharge (12%) or perianal/anal pain or discomfort
- Rectal gonorrhoea is a key marker for unprotected anal sex

Pharyngeal infection

- Typically asymptomatic (90%)

Conjunctival infection (adult)

- Uncommon, presents with unilateral or bilateral purulent discharge from one or both eyes and inflammation

Diagnosis

Diagnosis is made by detecting *N. gonorrhoeae* at an infected site. No test for gonorrhoea offers 100% sensitivity and specificity. Depending on the clinical setting and local factors (e.g. availability of tests, local prevalence of infection), there are three diagnostic tools.

NAATs

- are the test of choice for testing asymptomatic individuals for urethral or endocervical infection, and for testing rectal and pharyngeal infection in MSM
- have a high sensitivity (>96%) which is greater than culture
- in men a urethral sample or first void urine (FVU) are equally sensitive
- in women, urine is not the optimal specimen as this has lower sensitivity than both endocervical or vulvovaginal specimens which are equally sensitive
- are not licensed for extra-genital sites, therefore a reactive test from the pharynx or rectum should be confirmed by supplementary testing with a different nucleic acid target from the original test
- often offer testing for both chlamydia and gonorrhoea on the same specimen, a so-called 'dual NAAT test'

Microscopy

- A Gram-stained smear is examined by microscopy (magnification 1000×) to identify Gram-negative (stain light red) diplococci within PMNL (Figure 11.1)
- Not recommended for asymptomatic individuals as low sensitivity in these individuals
- Can be a useful near-patient test in specialist settings for men with urethral discharge (sensitivity good, approximately 95%) or women with endocervical discharge (poor sensitivity <50%), but only provides a provisional diagnosis
- Is not appropriate for pharyngeal specimens and has poor sensitivity for rectal specimens

Culture

- Is essential for monitoring antimicrobial sensitivity and emerging resistance, as antibiotic susceptibility testing can be carried out. A culture should therefore be taken in all cases of gonorrhoea diagnosed by NAATs prior to antibiotics being given (if possible)
- A specimen for culture should also be taken in symptomatic individuals (sample the symptomatic site, e.g. urethra, rectum, endocervix, throat), sexual contacts of individuals with gonorrhoea, individuals with suspected PID, or with any genital or rectal discharge
- Samples can be directly inoculated onto a culture medium (usually available in specialist settings) or collected in transport medium for later transfer to the laboratory
- If using a transport medium, specimens must be stored at 4°C (refrigerator) and transported within 48 hours of taking as *N. gonorrhoeae* has fastidious growth requirements and is susceptible to loss of viability if incorrect storage of specimens or delays in transport occurs
- Culture has high sensitivity (85–95%) and is cheap

Table 11.3 Causes of NGU

Infective causes
Chlamydia trachomatis 11 – 45%
Mycoplasma genitalium 10 – 25%
Trichomonas vaginalis 1 – 20%
Adenoviruses 2 – 4%
HSV 2 – 3%
Ureaplasma urealyticum
UTI may account for 6% of cases

Non-infective causes
Trauma, e.g. catheterization
Chemical irritation, e.g. spermicide cream, soap
Urethral stricture
Autoimmune disorder e.g. LS, Stevens–Johnson syndrome

Figure 11.2 Urethral discharge

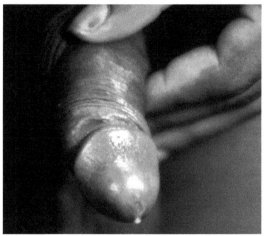

Source: CDC Public Health Image Library/Renelle Woodall.

Table 11.4 Recommended treatments for NGU*

Recommended treatments for NGU (including partners)
Azithromycin 1 g orally in a single dose
or
Doxycycline 100 mg twice a day orally for 7 days
Alternative regimens: Erythromycin 500 mg twice daily for 14 days
or
Ofloxacin 200 mg twice a day *or* 400 mg once a day for 7 days

Treatment for persistent/recurrent NGU
Azithromycin 500 mg stat orally, then 250 mg for 4 days plus metronidazole 400 mg b.d. for 5 days
or
Erythromycin 500 mg orally q.d.s. 21 days plus metronidazole 400 mg b.d. for 5 days

*For full list of treatment regimens please consult current BASHH guidance.

Figure 11.3 Gram-stained urethral smear showing 5 PMNLs per high-power field

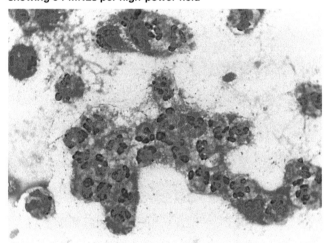

Source: Mark Mason, Senior Specialist Biomedical Scientist, Sandyford, NHS Greater Glasgow & Clyde, Glasgow, UK. Reproduced with permission of Sandyford.

Table 11.5 Relapsing NGU

Definition: Persistent or recurrent symptomatic urethritis occurring 30 – 90 days following treatment for acute NGU
Prevalence: Occurs in 10 – 20% of men treated for NGU
Treatment: (Table 11.4) should cover *M. genitalium* and *T. vaginalis*
Aetiology: Probably multifactorial. *M. genitalium* is implicated in 20 – 40% of cases. *M. genitalium* can be diagnosed by NAAT but this is not routinely available in the UK. It is a sexually transmitted organism and in addition to its role in NGU, it is likely to be responsible for at least some cases of urethritis, cervicitis and PID in women. *Ureaplasma urealyticum* and *Trichomonas vaginalis* have also been implicated.

Sites and timing of samples
- In asymptomatic men a FVU is collected and in asymptomatic women, a (self-taken) vulvovaginal swab for NAAT
- In men and women with symptoms, sample the relevant sites for NAAT and for culture
- The optimal testing period after exposure has not been established, although symptoms can appear within a few days. By convention testing for gonorrhoea is aligned with chlamydia testing, i.e. test at initial presentation and if the potential exposure is within the preceding 2 weeks, then retest 2 weeks after exposure

Complications
- PID, endometritis, epidiymo-orchitis, prostatitis
- Haematogenous dissemination (disseminated gonococcal infection – DGI) can cause skin lesions, arthralgia, arthritis and tenosynovitis although this is uncommon. DGI will rarely cause endocarditis and meningitis
- Neonatal gonococcal infection can occur due to exposure in the birth canal

Management

Treatment (Table 11.1)
Treatments for uncomplicated infections are listed in Table 11.1. Regimens for complicated infections, e.g. PID are given in the relevant chapters.

Resistance
Resistance of gonorrhoea to antibiotics has increased rapidly throughout the globe in recent years. High rates of resistance to tetracycline, penicillin and quinolone have been detected and these treatments are therefore not recommended in most countries (including the UK).

General
- Advise complete abstinence (no sexual contact even with a condom) until a negative TOC is obtained
- Give written information about the infection
- Offer screening for other STIs: testing for chlamydia should be undertaken routinely on all adults with gonorrhoea due to the high incidence of co-infection (41% of women and 35% of heterosexual men)
- Discuss consistent and correct use of barrier methods

Partner notification
- The "look-back" period for men with urethral symptoms is 2 weeks after development of the symptoms (or their last partner if longer)
- The 'look-back' period for asymptomatic infections or infections at other sites is 3 months

- Sexual partners should be offered testing and epidemiological treatment

Follow-up and TOC
- Follow-up after treatment is important to confirm adherence to treatment, and abstinence from sex
- Review antibiotic sensitivities if available
- TOC is recommended in all individuals
- If asymptomatic, test with a NAAT 2 weeks after completion of antibiotics (followed by culture if positive)
- If symptoms or signs persist, test with culture at least 72 hours after treatment completed
- If TOC is positive, this can be due to reinfection or may indicate antibiotic resistance

Non-gonococcal urethritis (NGU)
Urethritis is inflammation of the urethra. It is the commonest condition diagnosed and treated in men attending GUM clinics in the UK. Urethritis is described as NGU when *Neisseria gonorrhoeae* is not detected (and gonococcal when gonorrhoea is detected).

Aetiology
NGU is usually (but not always) sexually acquired. In at least 50% of men there is no identifiable pathogen. If an organism is isolated, the most common are *C. trachomatis* and *M. genitalium* (Table 11.3).

- Signs and symptoms: Urethral discharge, urethritis, dysuria, penile irritation (Figure 11.2)
- Complications: Epidiymo-orchitis, SARA (uncommon)
- Diagnosis and investigations: The diagnosis is made by microscopy. A Gram stained urethral smear examined by high power microscopy (×1000) should contain ≥5 PMNLs per microscopic field (Figure 11.3). Alternatively a centrifuged sample of first passed urine can be used (≥10 PMNL must be seen). Urethral smears are no longer taken from asymptomatic men. A NAAT for chlamydia and gonorrhoea should be taken ± a urethral culture for gonorrhoea. An MSSU should be sent if UTI is suspected. A full STI screen should be offered including HIV testing

Management
- General: Advise complete abstinence (no sexual contact even with a condom) until treatment is completed
- Treatment: should be initiated without waiting for results (Table 11.4)
- PN: Offer current partners screening and epidemiological treatment. 'Look back' period is 4 weeks
- Persistent/recurrent urethritis – Table 11.5

12 Vaginal discharge

Figure 12.1 Normal vaginal flora

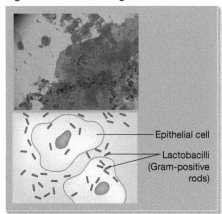

- Epithelial cell
- Lactobacilli (Gram-positive rods)

Source: Mark Mason, Senior Specialist Biomedical Scientist, Sandyford, NHS Greater Glasgow & Clyde, Glasgow, UK. Reproduced with permission of Sandyford.

Table 12.1 Causes of vaginal discharge

Infective, non-STI	Bacterial vaginosis (commonest) *Candida*
Infective, STI	*Chlamydia trachomatis* *Neisseria gonorrhoeae* *Trichomonas vaginalis* Herpes simplex virus
Non-infective causes	Physiological Cervical ectopy or polyp Foreign body (e.g. retained tampon) Malignancy of the genital tract Allergy or dermatitis Fistulae Associated with contraceptive method

Figure 12.3 Normal, < 4.5 (yellow) and raised > 4.5 (dark green) pH measurements

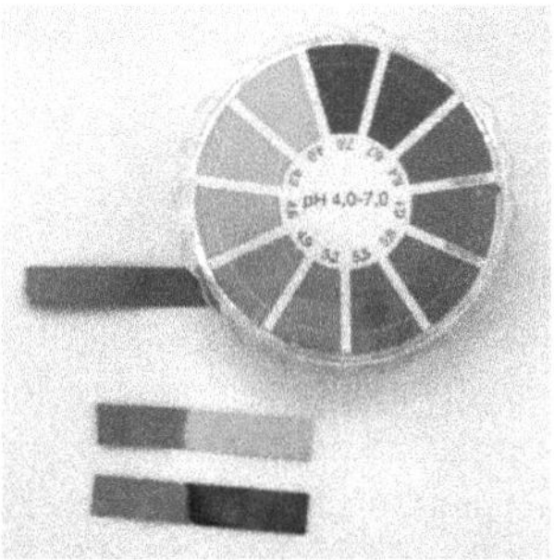

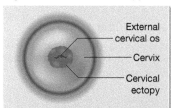

Figure 12.4 Cervical ectopy

- External cervical os
- Cervix
- Cervical ectopy

- A normal finding in women of reproductive age
- Due to eversion of the endocervix resulting in squamous metaplasia
- Women with cervical ectopy may complain of increased physiological discharge
- Characteristic red area surrounding the external os
- Ectopy can be treated with silver nitrate, or laser or cold coagulation after exclusion of cervical pathology
- There is a lack of evidence of the effectiveness of these treatments and they may initially worsen the discharge
- Exclusion of other causes and reassurance are often the best strategy

Box 12.1 Specific questions to ask about vaginal discharge

- Duration of symptoms
- Quantity of discharge
- Odour, colour, consistency
- Associated symptoms: vulval itch or soreness, irregular bleeding, pelvic or abdominal pain, dyspareunia, fever
- Does anything exacerbate the symptoms (e.g. menses, sexual intercourse) or improve them?
- Has the patient used any over-the-counter remedies (and did they help)?

Box 12.2 Factors affecting vaginal pH measurement

- Lubricant, e.g. KY jelly
- Semen
- Blood
- Cervical mucus

All these substances elevate the vaginal pH to > 4.5 (can mimic BV or TV)

Figure 12.2 Syndromic and empirical treatment

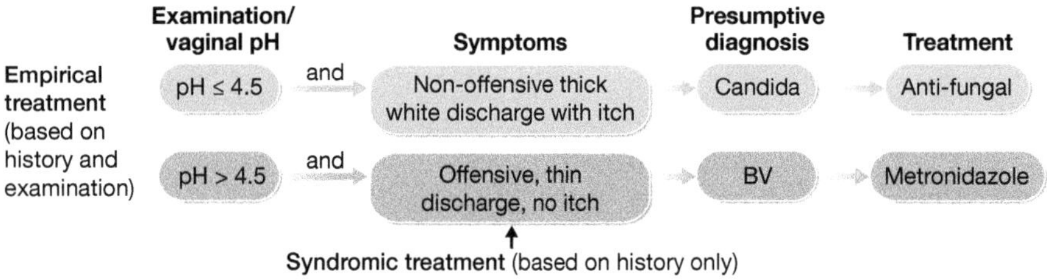

Examination/ vaginal pH	Symptoms	Presumptive diagnosis	Treatment
Empirical treatment (based on history and examination)	pH ≤ 4.5 and → Non-offensive thick white discharge with itch	Candida	Anti-fungal
	pH > 4.5 and → Offensive, thin discharge, no itch	BV	Metronidazole

↑ Syndromic treatment (based on history only)

Table 12.2 Features of normal and abnormal vaginal discharge

	Colour	Consistency and quantity	Odour	Associated symptoms	Vaginal pH	Diagnosis	Comments
Physiological	Clear, white	Varies (with menstrual cycle)	None	None	3.5 – 4.5	A diagnosis of exclusion	Normal finding
Bacterial vaginosis	Grey, milky, white	Watery, thin, profuse	Malodour (fishy)	None	> 4.5	Microscopy	Most common cause of abnormal discharge
Candida albicans	White	Thick, curd-like	None	Itch, soreness, swelling	3.5 – 4.5	Microscopy or culture	Often over-diagnosed
Trichomonas vaginalis*	Yellow	Thin, frothy, varies from scanty to profuse	Malodour (fishy)	Itch, irritation or soreness, dysuria	> 4.5	Microscopy or culture	Rarer than BV and *Candida* especially in the developed world
Chlamydia trachomatis*	Mucopurulent Bloodstained	Thick	None	PCB, IMB, abdominal pain	3.5 – 4.5	NAAT	70% women will be asymptomatic
Neisseria gonorrhoeae*	Mucopurulent Bloodstained	Thick	None	Abdominal pain, dysuria	3.5 – 4.5	NAAT (± microscopy and culture)	50% women will be asymptomatic

*These infections are sexually transmitted (STIs). See relevant chapters for management including partner notification

Sexual and Reproductive Health at a Glance, First Edition. Catriona Melville. © 2015 by John Wiley & Sons, Ltd. Published 2015 by John Wiley & Sons, Ltd.
Companion website: www.ataglanceseries.com/sexualhealth

Background

Vaginal discharge is a common presenting complaint in women of reproductive age. Abnormal vaginal discharge is a non-specific and subjective symptom. If a woman has underlying concerns regarding an STI, she may perceive a physiological discharge as abnormal.

The healthy vaginal environment

- The vagina is a dynamic ecosystem which is sterile at birth, becoming colonized within a few days with commensal bacteria (predominantly Gram-positive flora)
- The vaginal pH in premenarchal females is approximately neutral (pH 7.0)
- At puberty, the vaginal epithelium changes from cuboidal to stratified squamous. The predominant flora becomes lactobacilli (Figure 12.1), which metabolize glycogen in the vaginal epithelium to produce lactic acid. Thus the vaginal environment becomes acidic with a pH of ≤4.5
- Other commensals are found in the vagina in smaller amounts, e.g. *Candida albicans, Staphylococcus aureus* and *Streptococcus agalactiae* (Group B streptococcus). They can 'overgrow' and cause abnormal vaginal discharge

Vaginal discharge

- Physiological discharge is a normal finding in women of reproductive age and consists of desquamated epithelial cells from the vagina and cervix, mucus from the cervical glands, bacteria, and transudate from the vaginal wall. It is white in colour and non-offensive but the amount and type varies throughout the menstrual cycle
- An abnormal discharge can arise from anywhere in the genital tract, and may be due to infective or non-infective causes. Infections may be vaginal or cervical and can be sexually or non-sexually transmitted (Tables 12.1 and 12.2)

Infective causes

- Bacterial vaginosis (BV) is the most common cause of abnormal vaginal discharge in women of reproductive age but is often under-diagnosed
- Candida is also a common diagnosis in women but is often over-diagnosed
- TV usually presents with abnormal vaginal discharge but is much less common than either BV or candida
- Both chlamydia and gonorrhoea can present with abnormal vaginal discharge; however, chlamydia is asymptomatic in 70% women. If chlamydia is found in a woman with vaginal discharge this may be an incidental finding rather than the cause of the symptoms. Similarly many women with gonorrhoea are symptomless but up to half will present with abnormal vaginal discharge
- Herpes simplex virus (HSV) infection can cause cervicitis which occasionally presents as vaginal discharge. Additionally local inflammation associated with HSV infection can be accompanied by a vulval exudate which may present as vaginal discharge
- It is also important to consider that several pathologies can coexist, e.g. BV and chlamydia

History

- Take an appropriate clinical history including a sexual history to assess the STI risk
- Ask comprehensive questions about the nature of the vaginal discharge (Box 12.1), as this can point towards a likely diagnosis e.g. itch is associated with VVC but not BV
- Enquire about associated symptoms and specifically those indicative of upper reproductive tract infection

Examination

- If the patient has no symptoms suggestive of upper reproductive tract infection (PID), and is low risk for STIs an examination is not always essential particularly in non-specialist settings. If the examination is declined with such a history, then syndromic treatment may be given based on the clinical history alone (Figure 12.2)
- Women who present with failed treatment or recurrent symptoms should undergo an examination as should those who are pregnant, postpartum, post-abortion, or have undergone recent instrumentation of the genital tract

Vaginal pH

This simple and inexpensive test can help distinguish between the commonest causes of abnormal vaginal discharge namely BV and candida. Caution must be used when interpreting vaginal pH as it can be affected by 'contaminants' in the vagina (Box 12.2). Vaginal pH measurement (Figure 12.3) along with the clinical history can be useful to treat the patient empirically before the results of investigations are available (Figure 12.2).

Investigations

- STI testing should be offered to all sexually active women
- *Microscopy*: immediate wet mount and Gram stain microscopy can be used to identify TV, candida, BV and gonorrhoea. Specimens can be transferred to the laboratory for microscopy if onsite facilities do not exist however these are not as sensitive as immediate microscopy
- *NAAT testing*: for chlamydia and gonorrhoea should be undertaken by either an endocervical sample (if examining the woman) or a self-taken vulvo-vaginal swab
- *Endocervical swab*: this should be taken for culture and sensitivity testing if gonorrhoea is suspected. The sample can be directly plated onto culture medium or transported to the lab for delayed plating (see GC chapter for transport requirements)
- *High vaginal swabs (HVS)*: are often used in non-specialist settings and can be helpful for the diagnosis of BV, TV and candida, but may report commensals which can cause undue anxiety and overtreatment. BV may be under diagnosed with a HVS if additional criteria are not used. It is recommended that an HVS is reserved for those with failed treatment or recurrent symptoms, in women who are pregnant, post-partum or post-abortion, or have had recent instrumentation of the genital tract

Management

See Chapters 10, 11, 13, 14, and 15 for individual infections including management in pregnancy
- The clinical history and examination should be definitive in diagnosis of a retained foreign body, e.g. condom or tampon
- Cervical ectopy (Figure 12.4)

Contraception and vaginal discharge

- BV is more common in users of the Cu-IUD. COC or condom users have a reduced risk of BV. Women with recurrent BV who use the CU-IUD may consider switching to another method
- Although there is no clear evidence as to whether the use of hormonal contraception increases the risk of VVC, women using CHC methods may consider switching to another method
- The progestogen-only injectable may be associated with a reduced risk of BV and recurrent VVC

13 Bacterial vaginosis

Table 13.1 Vaginal pH and flora

Normal vaginal flora	pH 3.5 – 4.5	Lactobacilli predominate
Bacterial vaginosis	pH > 4.5	Anaerobic bacteria predominate

Box 13.1 Species of anaerobic bacteria associated with BV

Gardnerella vaginalis	*Atopobium vaginalis*
Prevotella spp.	*Clostridiales* spp.
Mycoplasma hominis	*Leptotrichia* spp.
Mobiluncus spp.	*Sneathia* spp.

Figure 13.1 Typical discharge seen with BV

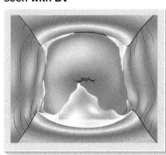

Figure 13.2 Gram-stained smear of a 'clue cell' seen in BV

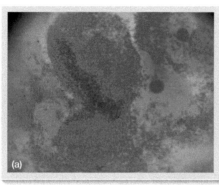

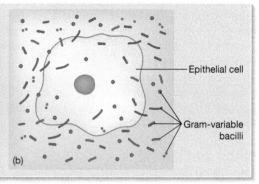

(a)   (b)

Epithelial cell

Gram-variable bacilli

Box 13.2 Amsel's criteria for diagnosis of BV

Three out of the following four criteria must be fulfilled:
• Thin, white, homogenous discharge
• 'Clue cells' seen on microscopy of a wet mount slide
• Vaginal pH > 4.5
• Positive amine test ('whiff test'): addition of 10% potassium hydroxide (KOH 10%) to vaginal fluid releases a fishy odour*

*Amine test is not widely used for safety reasons. KOH is caustic and potentially dangerous outside of a laboratory setting

Table 13.3 Treatments for BV

Recommended
Metronidazole 400 mg b.d. orally for 5 – 7 days
or Metronidazole 2 g in a single oral dose
or Intravaginal metronidazole gel (0.75%) once daily for 5 days
or Intravaginal clindamycin cream (2%) once daily for 7 days

Alternative
Tinidazole 2 g single oral dose
or Clindamycin 300 mg orally twice daily for 7 days
(risk of pseudomembranous colitis)

Pregnancy
Metronidazole 400 mg b.d. orally for 5 – 7 days

Recurrent BV
400 mg metronidazole orally twice daily for 3 days at start and/or end of menstruation
or 5 g 0.75% metronidazole gel intravaginally twice weekly for 16 weeks
or Lactic acid gel intravaginal for 3 days after menstruation for 6 months

Table 13.2 Hay/Ison criteria for appearance of vaginal flora on a Gram-stained smear

Grade	Appearance	Classification
Grade 1	Lactobacillus morphotypes predominate	Normal vaginal flora
Grade 2	A mixed bacterial flora with reduced number of lactobacilli and Gardnerella or Mobiluncus morphotypes also present	Intermediate flora
Grade 3	Few or absent lactobacilli; Gardnerella and/or Mobiluncus morphotypes predominate	BV flora

Background

Bacterial vaginosis (BV) is the commonest cause of abnormal vaginal discharge in women of reproductive age. The reported prevalence varies markedly depending on the population studied, e.g. 5% in a group of asymptomatic students to 50% of women in rural Uganda.

Aetiology
• BV is considered an imbalance of the normal vaginal flora
• BV is associated with an overgrowth of anaerobic bacteria and an increase in vaginal pH (Table 13.1 and Box 13.1)

• The vaginal ecosystem is a dynamic state and BV can remit and arise spontaneously in both sexually active and sexually inactive women
• BV is not thought to be sexually transmitted (although there is ongoing debate and research regarding this) but is associated with sexual activity in that it is linked with concurrent STIs and recent changes of sexual partner. It can however be found in virgins
• BV is associated with an increase risk of HIV acquisition
• An alkaline pH (>4.5) favours the growth of anaerobic bacteria which cause the symptoms of BV. Some women therefore find that factors which increase the vaginal pH, e.g. menstrual blood or semen (both alkaline), are associated with the onset of BV

Sexual and Reproductive Health at a Glance, First Edition. Catriona Melville. © 2015 by John Wiley & Sons, Ltd. Published 2015 by John Wiley & Sons, Ltd.
Companion website: www.ataglanceseries.com/sexualhealth

- The use of condoms, a circumcised partner and the COC appear to be protective against BV

Risk factors
- Black ethnicity, smoking, vaginal douching, receptive cunnilingus
- BV is more common in users of the Cu-IUD, although an association with the LNG-IUS is unclear

Symptoms and signs
- As many as 50% of women will have no symptoms
- Symptoms: moderate to profuse, offensive smelling vaginal discharge but usually no soreness or itch (although can coexist with VVC)
- Signs: Malodorous (fishy) grey or white discharge coating the vestibule and vaginal walls (Figure 13.1). Can 'pool' in the speculum if profuse and is sometimes frothy (c.f. TV). Usually no erythema or signs of inflammation

Diagnosis
pH measurement
This is a useful test which can be employed in specialist and non-specialist settings if the woman consents to an examination. BV is associated with an elevated vaginal pH of >4.5–6.0.

Microscopy
- The diagnosis of BV is based on the appearance of a vaginal smear on microscopy. Immediate microscopy is available in most specialized SRH settings. Alternatively a swab (HVS) or an air-dried slide can be transported to the local laboratory for Gram staining and microscopy
- There are two main diagnostic approaches; the Hay/Ison criteria and Amsel's criteria (Table 13.2 and Box 13.2)
- Clue cells (Figure 13.2) are vaginal epithelial cells covered in small Gram-variable bacilli (rods)

Culture
Gardnerella vaginalis can be cultured from the vagina of at least 50% of normal women therefore culture has **no** role in the diagnosis of BV.

   Commercially available tests: Point of care tests such as the OSOM BVblue test (which detects elevated levels of the enzyme sialidase), are not widely available in the UK, but perform adequately when compared to microscopy.

   NAATs: These are still under development and are being designed to detect combinations of BV associated bacteria.

Complications
- The prevalence of BV is high in women with PID but causality has not been demonstrated, and there have been no prospective studies to determine whether treating asymptomatic BV reduces the risk of developing subsequent PID
- BV is associated with postoperative vaginal cuff infection following transvaginal hysterectomy
- In one study BV was associated with NGU in male partners

Pregnancy
- BV is associated with late miscarriage, preterm rupture of the membranes (PROM), preterm birth and postpartum endometritis

- BV is associated with post-TOP endometritis and PID and therefore screening and/or antibiotic prophylaxis is recommended for women undergoing this procedure

Management
General
- Women should be advised to avoid perfumed shower gels and soaps coming into contact with the vulva/vagina; avoid bubble baths and vaginal douching
- Offer STI testing if appropriate as BV can co-exist with STIs

Treatment
- Indicated for symptomatic women, those undergoing certain surgical procedures (e.g. TOP), and for women who have no symptoms but choose to have treatment when offered
- Recommended and alternative treatment regimens are listed in Table 13.3
- The stat dose of metronidazole may be slightly less effective than the 5–7-day course, but cure rates with either of these regimens are 70–80%
- Alcohol must be avoided during metronidazole therapy and for 48 hours after completion
- The intravaginal therapies are more expensive than oral metronidazole and clindamycin cream weakens condoms
- *Allergy*: if allergic to metronidazole (uncommon), use clindamycin cream
- *Pregnancy*: see Table 13.3. There is insufficient evidence to recommend routine screening of pregnant women. Symptomatic pregnant women should be treated in the standard way. Vaginal preparations can be useful in breastfeeding women to avoid altering the taste of breast milk

Partner notification
- Treating male partners of women with BV does not affect the relapse rate, therefore is not indicated
- Not yet established whether treating female partners of women with BV has any value

Follow up and TOC
- Not required if symptoms have resolved

Recurrent BV
- Up to 30% of women will have a recurrence within 3 months of treatment although the cause is unknown. It may be that the normal vaginal flora have not full re-established. Some women have frequent recurrences
- The diagnosis should be confirmed with microscopy
- Good genital hygiene practices should be reiterated (e.g. stop douching)
- If the women uses an IUD for contraception, an alternative method may need to be considered
- There is insufficient evidence supporting the use of vaginal acidifying gels, e.g. Relactagel® or Balance Activ®, however these are anecdotally useful
- Probiotic therapy may also be useful

14 Vulvovaginal candidiasis

Figure 14.1 Typical curd-like adherent discharge seen in VVC

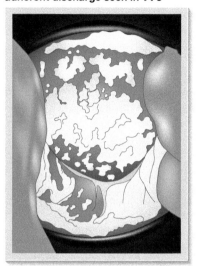

Figure 14.2 Microscopic appearance of *C. albicans* on Gram stain

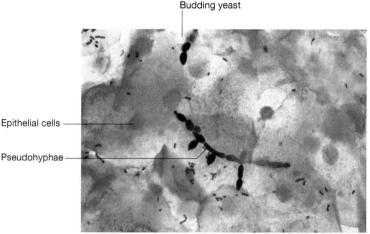

Budding yeast

Epithelial cells

Pseudohyphae

Source: Mark Mason, Senior Specialist Biomedical Scientist, Sandyford, NHS Greater Glasgow & Clyde, Glasgow, UK. Reproduced with permission of Sandyford.

Table 14.1 Treatment for uncomplicated VVC

Oral

- Fluconazole 150 mg stat dose ⎤ Avoid in pregnancy
- Itraconozole 200 mg b.d. for 1 day ⎦ and breastfeeding

Vaginal*

- Clotrimazole 500 mg pessary stat
- Clotrimazole vaginal cream (10%) 5 g stat at night
- Clotrimazole pessary 100 mg 6 nights
- Clotrimazole pessary 200 mg 3 nights
- Miconazole nitrate 2% cream with applicators once daily for 10 – 14 days or twice daily for 7 days
- Miconazole nitrate 1.2 g ovule stat dose at night
- Econazole nitrate 150 mg pessary 3 nights
- Econazole nitrate 150 mg pessary stat dose
- Fenticonazole nitrate cream 2% insert 5 g twice daily for 3 days
- Fenticonazole nitrate 200 mg capsule 3 nights
- Fenticonazole nitrate 600 mg capsule stat dose at night

Combined*

- Clotrimazole (10%) vaginal cream with applicator and 2% topical cream
- Clotrimazole 500 g pessary and 2% topical cream

Topical* (in addition to oral or vaginal for vulval symptoms)

- Clotrimazole cream 1% 2 – 3 times daily
- Clotrimazole cream 2% 2 – 3 times daily
- Econazole nitrate 1% cream 14 nights
- Ketoconozole cream 2% once or twice daily

*Latex condoms and diaphragms may be damaged by vaginal or topical preparations containing econazole, miconazole, isoconazole, fenticonazole or clotrimazole

Table 14.2 Treatment for recurrent VVC

Induction

*Fluconazole oral capsule 150 mg every 72 hours 3 doses

Maintenance

*Fluconazole oral capsule 150 mg once a week for 6 months

Alternative options for maintenance

†Clotrimazole pessary 500 mg once a week
*Fluconazole oral capsule 50 mg daily
*Itraconazole oral capsule 50 – 100 mg daily
*Ketoconazole oral capsule 100 mg daily

*Avoid in pregnancy and breastfeeding
†May damage latex barrier methods

Sexual and Reproductive Health at a Glance, First Edition. Catriona Melville. © 2015 by John Wiley & Sons, Ltd. Published 2015 by John Wiley & Sons, Ltd.
Companion website: www.ataglanceseries.com/sexualhealth

Background

Vulvovaginal candidiasis (VVC) is common in women of reproductive age. It is estimated that 75% of women will have at least one episode of symptomatic VVC in their lifetime.

- *Aetiology:* In 80–92% of cases VVC is caused by the yeast *Candida albicans*. The remaining episodes are caused by non-albicans species such as *C. glabrata*, *C. tropicalis* or *C. krusei*
- 10–20% of women have vaginal colonization with *Candida* sp. and therefore in the absence of symptoms the isolation of candida does not require treatment
- It is not an STI
- VVC is associated with vaginal exposure to estrogen and therefore symptomatic VVC is uncommon before the menarche and after the menopause but is common in the reproductive years and pregnancy
- Predisposing host factors include diabetes, immunosuppression, antimicrobial therapy (causes disturbance of vaginal flora and increase yeast carriage) and vulval irritation/trauma
- VVC is mostly uncomplicated and responds to simple treatment; however, candidiasis in pregnancy, recurrent episodes, VVC caused by non-albicans species or abnormal host factors (e.g. diabetes) can be more challenging to manage

Symptoms and signs

- Symptoms: vulva itch, irritation or soreness; external dysuria, superficial dyspareunia, vaginal discharge
- Signs: vulval erythema (vulvovaginitis), oedema, fissuring, satellite lesions, excoriation, discharge
- Vaginal discharge occurs in 50% of women with VVC. It is non-offensive and typically curdy. On examination it adheres to the vaginal walls in white plaques (Figure 14.1)

Diagnosis

Women are often treated empirically in non-specialist settings on the basis of the history (see Chapter 12 Figure 12.2). If symptoms persist or reoccur, examination and further investigations are indicated. Vaginal pH measurement can be helpful in distinguishing VVC from other diagnoses. The vaginal pH remains normal with a pH 4.0–4.5.

Microscopy

- A lateral vaginal wall sample can be prepared as a wet mount and/or a Gram stain
- Immediate microscopy of a Gram stain can demonstrate pseudohyphae and spores in 65% of symptomatic women with symptoms of candidiasis (Figure 14.2)
- The sensitivity of a wet mount slide (saline microscopy) of vaginal discharge in symptomatic women is 40–60%

Culture

- This remains the gold standard for diagnosis of candida
- It is useful if microscopy is inconclusive or if identification of the species type is important, e.g. in recurrent VVC
- A specimen can either be plated directly onto culture medium (e.g. Sabouraud's) or transported to the laboratory in transport medium (i.e. a HVS) for delayed inoculation
- Culture has a sensitivity of 70–80% and a specificity of >99%

Management

General

General genital hygiene advice should be given to women suffering from VVC:

- Local irritants, e.g. perfumed soaps and wipes, should be avoided
- An emollient can be used as a soap substitute
- Wear cotton underwear and loose fitting clothes

Treatments

- Either intravaginal or oral azole treatments can be used as both have similar efficacy (>80% cure rate)
- Table 14.1 lists examples of the available treatments. For a comprehensive list consult the British National Formulary (BNF)
- Personal preference, cost and availability will determine choice of preparation
- Topical agents can be used in addition to oral or intravaginal treatments for women with vulval symptoms but there is little evidence that this will have any advantage over the use of an emollient and it has the potential to cause a local irritant reaction

Follow-up and PIN

Follow-up and test of cure are not required if symptoms resolve. There is no indication to screen or treat asymptomatic sexual partners of women with (either episodic or recurrent) VVC.

VVC in pregnancy

- Symptomatic VVC is common during pregnancy
- Asymptomatic colonization with Candida species is also more prevalent during pregnancy (30–40%)
- There is no association with adverse pregnancy outcomes
- Treatment of symptomatic VVC should be with topical imidazoles (e.g. clotrimazole). Longer courses of treatment may be required, e.g. 7 days
- Oral treatments are contraindicated due to unknown teratogenic effect

Recurrent VVC

- *Definition:* four or more episodes of symptomatic VVC in 12 months (at least two mycologically proven)
- Approximately 5% of women with a primary episode of VVC will develop recurrent disease
- Usually due to *C. albicans* rather than non-albicans species
- *Pathogenesis:* this is poorly understood, but host factors are implicated especially poorly controlled diabetes, immunosuppression and the use of broad spectrum antibiotics
- *Contraception:* COCs were implicated historically but modern combined methods contain low doses of estrogen and there is no clear evidence that they increase the risk of VVC. There is some evidence that the injectable progestogen may reduce the likelihood of recurrent disease due to relative hypoestrogenism
- *Investigations:* if indicated by the history, a random blood glucose should be taken. Culture with speciation and sensitivities should be requested to exclude non-albicans species
- *Management:* general advice should be the same as with a primary episode. An induction and maintenance regimen should be used for 6 months (Table 14.2); 90% of women remain disease-free during treatment however this declines to 40% at 1 year
- *Alternative treatments:* there is insufficient evidence to support the use of oral or vaginal lactobacillus, changes to diet or the use of tee tree oil in the prevention of VVC

15 Trichomonas vaginalis

Figure 15.1 Vaginal discharge typical with TV

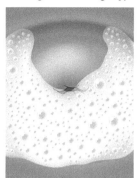

Figure 15.2 Strawberry cervix

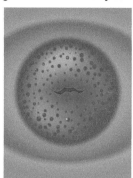

Figure 15.3 Narrow range pH paper

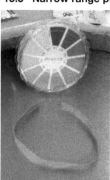

Figure 15.4 Trichomonads on microscopy

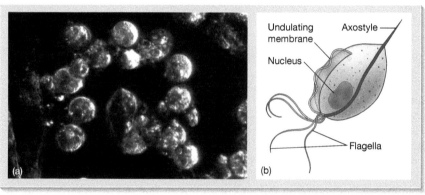

Source: Mark Mason, Senior Specialist Biomedical Scientist, Sandyford, NHS Greater Glasgow & Clyde, Glasgow, UK.
Reproduced with permission of Sandyford.

Figure 15.5 Recurrent or relapsing TV

Causes: non-adherence to treatment, partners not treated, re-infection, poor absorption of drug or vomiting

Management
- Check compliance and confirm that partner has been treated and they have abstained from sexual contact
- Patients often respond to a second course of standard treatment even when the first course has failed
- Some organisms present in the vagina may interact with nitroimidazoles and reduce their effectiveness therefore the use of a broad spectrum antibiotic e.g. erythromycin before retreating with metronidazole has been recommended
- Management of metronidazole-resistant TV is a therapeutic challenge. Higher doses of metronidazole can be used if standard re-treatment fails, e.g.
  Metronidazole 400 mg t.d.s. orally 7 days
  plus
  Metronidazole 1 g PR or PV (unlicensed) daily for 7 days
  or
  Metronidazole 2 g daily orally for 3 to 5 days

For a full list of current recommended treatment options refer to BASHH guidance

Background

Trichomoniasis is the most prevalent non-viral STI worldwide, with an estimated 276.4 million new diagnoses in 2008 (WHO). It is most prevalent in developing countries whereas there has been a steady decline in diagnoses in developed countries. In the UK diagnoses of trichomoniasis account for about 2% of GUM clinic attendances.

- Aetiology: trichomoniasis is a curable STI caused by the flagellated protozoal parasite *Trichomonas vaginalis* (TV)

- Transmission: in adults, TV is almost exclusively sexually transmitted. It is a site-specific infection and requires direct inoculation of the organism
- Female to female transmission can occur
- Sites of infection: in women the organism is found in the vagina, urethra and periurethral glands. In men, it mainly infects the urethra but has also been isolated from the subpreputial sac

Sexual and Reproductive Health at a Glance, First Edition. Catriona Melville. © 2015 by John Wiley & Sons, Ltd. Published 2015 by John Wiley & Sons, Ltd.
Companion website: www.ataglanceseries.com/sexualhealth

- TV is associated with an increased risk of HIV acquisition and is also associated with other STIs, e.g. *N. gonorrhoeae*
- TV has a spontaneous cure rate of 20–25%

Symptoms and signs (Figures 15.1, 15.2)

Females

- 10–50% of women are asymptomatic
- *Symptoms*: Profuse, offensive vaginal discharge (in up to 70%), dysuria, vulval soreness or itching
- *Signs*: 5–15% will have no signs on examination; 10–30% will have profuse frothy yellow malodorous vaginal discharge; vulvovaginitis; 2% will have strawberry cervix (small punctuate cervical haemorrhages with ulceration)

Males

- 15–50% asymptomatic – men often present as partners of women with TV
- *Symptoms*: urethral discharge, dysuria, frequency
- *Signs*: often none but may see urethral discharge and rarely balanoposthitis

Diagnosis

This will depend on the clinical setting and availability of tests e.g. near patient microscopy.

Investigations in females

- Vaginal pH measurement: this is a simple point-of-care investigation which can be done in most clinical settings. A sample is taken from the lateral vaginal wall and placed on narrow range pH paper (Figure 15.3). TV is associated with an elevated vaginal pH of >4.5
- Microscopy: motile trichomonads can be observed via immediate microscopy of a specimen taken from the posterior vaginal fornix (Figure 15.4). The slide is prepared as a 'wet mount' (suspended in saline). Motility will diminish with time. This investigation has a sensitivity of 40–80%
- High vaginal swab: this sample can be taken where immediate microscopy is unavailable. It must be transported to the laboratory as soon as possible (within 6 hours)
- Culture: TV specific culture will diagnose up to 95%, but not all laboratories offer this
- NAAT: these are not widely available or used yet

Investigations in men

- Identification of the organism in males is difficult so treatment is often epidemiological
- Microscopy: a urethral smear can be prepared in saline for immediate microscopy but the sensitivity is only 30%
- Culture: a urethral specimen or first void urine sample (ideally centrifuged within the hour) can be used for culture. Doing both together will significantly increase the diagnostic rate

Liquid-based cervical cytology

- TV can be found on cervical cytology samples as an incidental finding

- There can be a high false positive rate (up to 30%) therefore the diagnosis should be confirmed by culture or microscopy before treatment

Complications

- *Pregnancy*: infection with TV may be associated with pre-term rupture of the membranes, preterm delivery and low birth weight, but further research is required to confirm a causal relationship

Management

General

- Advise complete abstinence (no sexual contact even with a condom) until the individual and their partner have been treated
- Give written information about the infection
- Offer screening for other STIs
- Discuss consistent and correct use of barrier methods

Treatment

Most strains of *T. vaginalis* are highly susceptible to nitroimidazole drugs (95% cure rate). Recommended regimens:

- Metronidazole 2 g orally in a single dose

or

- Metronidazole 400–500 mg twice daily for 5–7 days

Alcohol should be avoided for the duration of treatment and for 48 hours thereafter due to possibility of a disulfiram-like reaction.

Treatment in pregnancy

- There is no evidence that metronidazole is a teratogenic drug. The BNF advises against high dose regimens in pregnancy. The drug enters breast milk and can alter the taste therefore high dose regimens should also be avoided in breastfeeding women
- Metronidazole 400 mg b.d. for 5–7 days is recommended in pregnancy or breastfeeding

Partner notification

- Current partners should be treated regardless of their test results
- Sexual contacts in the 4 weeks prior to presentation should be treated
- Partners should be offered STI screening

Follow-up/TOC

- At 2 weeks, follow-up is useful to determine resolution of symptoms, confirm compliance with treatment and abstinence from sexual contact and to complete PN
- If still symptomatic then a test of cure should be arranged (microscopy or culture) but this is not indicated if symptoms have resolved
- At 2 weeks, repeat urethral microscopy should be performed on men who were found to have an excess of polymorphs on initial microscopy to assess whether further treatment for non-gonococcal urethritis (NGU) is required
- Recurrent/relapsing TV can be challenging (Figure 15.5)

16 Syphilis

Table 16.1 Classification of syphilis

Acquired	Early (infectious syphilis; first 2 years of infection)	Primary	
		Secondary	
		Early latent	
	Late syphilis (after 2 years of infection)	Late latent	No signs or symptoms; positive serology
		Gummatous Cardiovascular Neurological	Symptomatic late syphilis (or known as tertiary syphilis but this definition generally excludes meningovascular syphilis)
Congenital	Early	Diagnosed within first 2 years of life	
	Late	Presents after 2 years	

Box 16.1 Genital ulcer prompt

Any anogenital ulcer should be considered syphilis until proven otherwise

Box 16.2 Argyll Robertson pupils

Argyll Robertson pupils

(usually) bilateral small irregular pupils that constrict to accommodation but not to light

Figure 16.2 Clinical features of symptomatic late syphilis

Neurosyphilis
- Asymptomatic: abnormal CSF findings; no signs or symptoms; uncertain significance
- Meningovascular: facial arteritis → infarction/meningeal inflammation, e.g. hemiplegia, paresis, seizures. Frequent pupillary abnormalities, e.g. Argyll Robertson pupils
- Tabes dorsalis: inflammation of spinal dorsal column → lightning pains, paraesthesia, areflexia, sensory ataxia, Charcot's joints (neuropathic joints)
- General paresis: cortical neuronal loss → gradual decline in cognitive functions and memory, personality change (antisocial), dementia, psychosis

Box 16.3 Hutchinson's triad (found in late congenital syphilis)

Hutchinson's incisors   Interstitial keratitis

Eighth nerve deafness

Figure 16.1 Primary syphilis

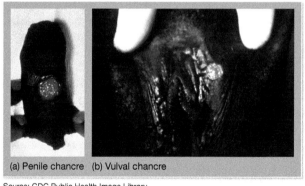

(a) Penile chancre   (b) Vulval chancre

Source: CDC Public Health Image Library

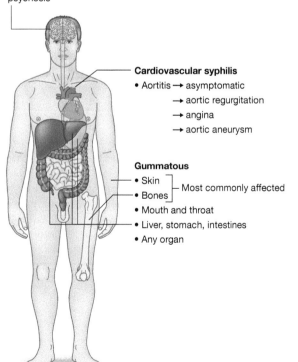

Cardiovascular syphilis
- Aortitis → asymptomatic
  - → aortic regurgitation
  - → angina
  - → aortic aneurysm

Gummatous
- Skin ⎤
- Bones ⎦ Most commonly affected
- Mouth and throat
- Liver, stomach, intestines
- Any organ

Figure 16.3 Dental malformations in congenital syphilis

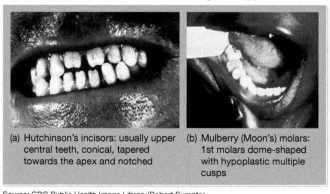

(a) Hutchinson's incisors: usually upper central teeth, conical, tapered towards the apex and notched

(b) Mulberry (Moon's) molars: 1st molars dome-shaped with hypoplastic multiple cusps

Source: CDC Public Health Image Library/Robert Sumpter

Sexual and Reproductive Health at a Glance, First Edition. Catriona Melville. © 2015 by John Wiley & Sons, Ltd. Published 2015 by John Wiley & Sons, Ltd.
Companion website: www.ataglanceseries.com/sexualhealth

Background

The WHO estimated there were 10.6 million cases of this curable sexually transmitted genital ulcerative infection diagnosed worldwide in 2008. It remains a significant health problem in both the USA and in Europe. Following a sharp decline in incidence in the UK in the 1980s, the number of cases increased rapidly between 1998 and 2008. In the UK there are a disproportionate number of cases in MSM and the majority of infections are in people >25 years of age, although recent outbreaks in young heterosexuals have been reported. Generally diagnoses in men far outweigh those in women but this is predominantly due to the high incidence in MSM. Surveillance data are collected on early infectious syphilis in the UK, USA and other countries.

- Aetiology: syphilis is caused by infection with the spirochete bacterium *Treponema pallidum* subsp. *pallidum* (other subspecies cause Yaws and Pinta). It has limited viability out with its host (obligate human parasite)
- Transmission: syphilis is transmitted by direct contact with an infectious lesion (usually sexual); via infected blood products or needle sharing; or vertical transmission (mother to child) as it can cross the placenta at any stage of pregnancy. Sexual transmission can be via the anogenital or oral contact
- Classification (Table 16.1)

Clinical features

Primary syphilis

- Characterized by a chancre (ulcer) which is typically solitary, indurated and painless, with a clean moist base, exuding clear serum (Figure 16.1). The chancre is typically in the anogenital region
- Atypical presentation can occur with ulcers which are multiple, painful, purulent or destructive and can mimic HSV infection (Box 16.1). They can also be extragenital, especially oral and rarely finger, hand, arm and other sites. Balanitis of Follman is rarely reported
- The primary lesion is associated with regional lymphadenopathy
- Occurs 9–90 days after infection (average is 3 weeks) and resolves within 3–8 weeks. May go unnoticed by the patient particularly if painless

Secondary syphilis

Haematogenous dissemination of infection causes multisystem involvement within the first 2 years of infection. Features are:
- Rash: generalized macular, papular or maculo-papular, often affecting the palms and soles. Classically the rash is non-itchy but can be associated with itch especially in patients with dark skin
- Condylomata lata: papular wart-like lesions located on moist areas especially around the vulva and anus
- 80% of patients will have skin lesions (rash, condylomata lata)
- Lymphadenopathy: inguinal or generalized (in 60% patients)
- Mucous membrane lesions in oral cavity, larynx or anogenital areas (in 30% of patients). Ulcers have a white border and can coalesce with other lesions forming "snail track" ulcers
- Less commonly (<10% of patients): patchy alopecia, anterior uveitis, splenomegaly, hepatitis, glomerulonephritis, periostitis, meningitis and cranial nerve palsies

Latent syphilis

Definition: positive serology for *T. Pallidum* with no signs or symptoms. If within first 2 years of infection it is classified as early latent disease. Thereafter it is defined as late latent syphilis.

Symptomatic late syphilis (Figure 16.2, Box 16.2)

Occurs > 2 years after initial infection. Untreated syphilis will progress to this symptomatic stage in approximately one-third of patients
- Gummatous: average onset after infection is 15 years, although can occur more than 40 years after initial infection. Gumma are destructive granulomatous nodular lesions due to reactivation of residual treponemes. They are not contagious. Lesions affect the musculo-skeletal, visceral and mucosal systems
- Cardiovascular syphilis: typically occurs 10–30 years after infection
- Neurosyphilis: can be further defined as asymptomatic (can occur early or late in the disease), tabes dorsalis (occurs 15–25 years after infection), general paresis (occurs 10–20 years after infection), and meningovascular neurosyphilis (occurs 2–7 years after infection). There is significant overlap in the spectrum of neurological disease

Congenital syphilis

Early: First 2 years of life
- Failure to thrive
- Mucosal lesions: snuffles, haemorrhagic rhinitis, progresses to local destruction (nasal cartilage) and perforation
- Skin: rash (especially around the mouth and body orifices), blistering bullous lesions (syphilitic pemphigus) condylomata lata around anus and genitalia
- Generalized lymphadenopathy and hepatosplenomegaly
- Bone: osteochondritis, periostitis pseudoparalysis
- Other; haemolysis and thrombocytopenia, neurological and ocular involvement, glomerulonephritis

Late: after 2 years of age. 60% will have no clinical features and be diagnosed on serology.
Malformations:
- Craniofacial: frontal bossing, short maxilla, high palatal arch, protuberance of mandible, saddlenose deformity, circumoral rhagades (fissures or linear scars in the skin)
- Dental: Hutchinson's incisors, Mulberry (Moon's) molars (Figure 16.3 and Box 16.3)
- Skeletal: bony sclerosis or nodules mainly of long bones, e.g. Sabre tibia
Inflammation:
- Interstitial keratitis (Box 16.3)
- Deafness (Box 16.3)
- Clutton's joints: bilateral painless effusion, usually of the knee joints
- Other: paroxysmal cold haemoglobinuria, neurological or gummatous involvement

Diagnosis

A thorough clinical history and examination should be undertaken looking for the above features. Indicators of possible infection should be sought from the history, e.g. an obstetric history of stillbirths or miscarriages. Particular attention should be given to examining the genitals, skin and lymph nodes for signs of primary and secondary syphilis if early infection is suspected. If late or congenital syphilis is suspected, examination of all systems is necessary.

Figure 16.4 Dark ground microscopy

Preparation of specimen

- Clean ulcer with a swab soaked in sterile saline
- Release serum by gently squeezing the ulcer
- Collect serum with the edge of a coverslip and mount in normal saline
- Cover with a coverslip and examine immediately (within 20 minutes)

T. pallidum on dark ground microscopy

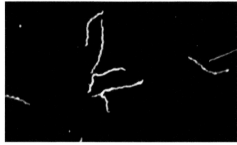

Source: Mark Mason, Senior Specialist Biomedical Scientist, Sandyford,
NHS Greater Glasgow & Clyde, Glasgow, UK. Reproduced with permission of Sandyford.

Table 16.3 Causes of biological false-positive reactions with syphilis serology

Biological false-positive reactions (BFPR) with cardiolipin tests (e.g. VDRL/RPR) occur in < 1% of the population and can be:	**Acute** • disappears within 6 months; usually in younger individuals (< 30 years) *or*	• Pregnancy • Vaccination • Acute febrile illnesses, e.g. chicken pox, viral hepatitis, atypical pneumonia, LGV, infectious mononucleosis
	Chronic • positive indefinitely; associated with aging (> 30 years)	• Autoimmune or connective tissue diseases, e.g. SLE, rheumatoid arthritis • Chronic infections, e.g. leprosy • Drug addiction (narcotic)

Table 16.2 Syphilis serology

Syphilis serology	Name of test	Abbreviation	Purpose	Benefits	Disadvantages/limitations
Specific (for anti-treponemal antibodies) tests	Treponemal enzyme immunoassay (EIA) to detect immunoglobulin G (IgG), immunoglobulin M (IgM) or both	EIA-IgG EIA-IgM EIA-IgG and IgM	• Screening and confirmation • IgM detectable towards end of week 2 post-infection • IgG detectable in week 4 or 5 post-infection	• Invariably positive in secondary and early latent syphilis	• Antibody titres correlate poorly with disease activity therefore tests are not used to assess response to treatment or re-infection • Do not differentiate between venereal syphilis and endemic syphilis (yaws and pinta)
	T. pallidum particle agglutination assay	TPPA	Screening and confirmation	TPPA is preferred to TPHA as is it more sensitive in primary infection	• TPPA titre does not correlate with disease activity or response
	T. pallidum haemagglutination assay (TPHA)	TPHA	Screening and confirmation		
	Fluorescent treponemal antibody absorbed test	FTA-abs	Historical confirmatory test, though not recommended as standard confirmatory test		
Non-specific tests (non-treponemal, or cardiolipin antigen tests)	Venereal disease research laboratory slide test	VDRL	Monitoring the response to treatment using serial titres	• Rapid, simple, inexpensive • Useful in assessing serial titres (quantitative test)	• Biological false-positive results (Table 16.3) • False-negative results: the prozone phenomenon • Poor sensitivity in late syphilis
	Rapid plasma reagin test	RPR			

Investigations

Testing for syphilis should always include serology. In addition if there are suspicious lesions then dark ground microscopy and PCR should be performed where available.

Dark ground microscopy

- Also known as dark field microscopy, this is an illumination technique whereby the object is lit by oblique rays of light. It is used for viewing unstained samples and causes them to appear brightly lit against a dark (almost black) background
- Dark ground microscopy demonstrates *T. Pallidum* directly but is not of value in intra-anal or oral lesions (as contamination with other commensal treponemes is likely)
- Specimens: serous exudates from any visible chancres/ulcers should be collected in primary syphilis (Figure 16.4), or from mucous patches or condylomata lata in secondary syphilis. Alternatively, regional lymph nodes can be aspirated to obtain a specimen
- Treponemes will be seen as tight spiral bacteria with rotator cork-screw like motility and angulation where the treponemes bend to almost 90° near their centres (Figure 16.4)
- If a lesion is suspicious but dark ground microscopy is negative, then this should be repeated one week later

NAAT-PCR

- A swab from an ulcer can be sent in viral transport medium for PCR. Some laboratories use a combined PCR test for *T. Pallidum* and HSV 1 and 2
- PCR has a high sensitivity (95%) and specificity (99%) for primary syphilis
- PCR has limited availability in many services and the result is not available immediately, so it should not replace dark ground microscopy, rather be done alongside it if available
- It is useful for non-genital (especially oral) lesions as there is no interference by commensals

Serology

Up to 15% of individuals with primary syphilis will be seronegative at initial presentation. Serology is usually positive at 4 weeks after infection but can take up to 3 months. There are two main types of serological test; specific and non-specific (Table 16.2).

- Specific (treponemal tests) tests: TPPA, Treponemal IgG/IgM and Inno-LIA. Treponemal antibody tests (except IgM) often remain positive for life
- Non-specific: VDRL and RPR are important for monitoring response to treatment. They eventually become non-reactive after treatment
In the UK a highly sensitive test is used for screening, e.g. EIA IgG/IgM or TPPA, and this is followed by a highly sensitive and specific confirmatory test (different from the initial test) e.g. TPPA or TPHA. The choice of screening test varies locally and in different countries but most will employ an initial screening test followed by a confirmatory test. Further testing may be done in a regional laboratory.
- **Prozone phenomenon** (cardiolipin tests): occurs in up to 2% of infected individuals and refers to a false negative result from strongly positive samples due to overwhelming antibody titres. It is most commonly associated with secondary syphilis and also more common in HIV-infected individuals. It can be overcome by appropriate serum dilutions
- All positive tests should be repeated on a second specimen for confirmation. False positives can occur (Table 16.3)
- Rapid point of care tests are available but mainly of use in outreach or field conditions in developing countries

Additional investigations

- A full STI screen including HIV testing should be offered
- The following investigations may be indicated depending on symptoms and examination findings: CXR, ECG (refer to cardiologist if features of CVS syphilis) lumbar puncture for examination of CSF (not recommended if asymptomatic and no signs of neurosyphilis), neurological imaging if neurological symptoms or signs (e.g. CT/MRI), biopsy and histology of gummatous lesions (although usually diagnosed clinically), X-ray to assess skeletal involvement
- Congenital syphilis: PCR or dark ground microscopy of exudates can be undertaken to demonstrate *T. pallidum*. Serological tests on infant's (not cord) blood; however, IgG crosses the placenta so this may be positive due to maternal antibodies. Demonstration of IgM is important but this can take up to 3 months to appear and should therefore be repeated (at 3, 6, and 12 months) if initially negative and other tests are reactive. Diagnosis is confirmed on serology by a positive IgM EIA test and/or a sustained VDRL/RPR or TPPA titre >4 times the maternal level. If the diagnosis is confirmed, further neonatal investigations are indicated, e.g. FBC, LFT, CSF examination, X-rays of long bones and ophthalmic assessment

Syphilis and HIV co-infection

- The risk of HIV acquisition increases in the presence of infectious syphilis and syphilis facilitates the transmission of HIV. Testing for HIV is recommended as the infections often coexist
- Clinical features in HIV-positive and negative individuals with early syphilis may be similar however HIV-infected individuals may present with large /multiple or deeper genital ulcers
- HIV-infected individuals with early syphilis may have an increased risk of neurological complications
- Serological tests in patients with HIV co-infection are generally reliable although false negative tests and delayed appearance of seroreactivity has been reported. The RPR/VDRL titre tends to be lower in primary syphilis and significantly higher in secondary disease in individuals with HIV infection
- A lumbar puncture is recommended in all HIV positive patients with neurological or ophthalmological signs/symptoms, if the VDRL is ≥1:32 at any stage or if there is treatment failure
- Treatment should be the same as for non-HIV infected individuals at each stage of infection. Some clinicians will offer HIV-positive individuals the option of a neurosyphilis treatment course whatever their infection stage, but evidence is lacking regarding this
- HIV co-infected patients should be followed up for life with 6 monthly serology (3 monthly in an outbreak situation)

Table 16.4 Treatment for syphilis

Clinical stage	Recommended regimens	Alternative regimens e.g. penicillin allergy or refusal of parenteral treatment	Notes
Incubating syphilis/ epidemiological treatment	Benzathine penicillin G 2.4 MU i.m. stat	Doxycycline 100 mg b.d. for 14 days orally	Steroid cover should be given when treating cardiovascular syphilis and neurosyphilis, e.g. prednisolone 40 – 60 mg daily orally for 3 days starting 24 hours prior to commencement of anti-treponemal therapy
Early syphilis	Benzathine penicillin G 2.4 MU i.m. stat *or* Procaine penicillin G 600 mg (600 000 units) i.m. daily for 10 days	Doxycycline 100 mg b.d. for 14 days orally *or* Erythromycin 500 mg orally q.d.s. for 14 days *or* Ceftriaxone 500 mg i.m. daily for 10 days (if no penicillin anaphylaxis)	
Late latent, CVS and gummatous	Benzathine penicillin G 2.4 MU i.m. weekly for 2 weeks (3 doses on days 1, 8 and 15) *or* Procaine penicillin G 600 mg (600 000 units) i.m. once daily for 17 days	Doxycycline 100 mg b.d. orally for 28 days	
Neurosyphilis	Procaine penicillin G 1.8 – 2.4 MU i.m. daily plus probenacid 500 mg q.d.s. orally for 17 days *or* Benzyl penicillin 18 – 24 MU daily given as 3 – 4 MU IV every 4 – 6 hours for 17 days	Doxycycline 200 mg b.d. orally for 28 days *or* Amoxicillin 2 g t.d.s. orally plus probenacid 500 mg q.d.s orally for 28 days	
Early syphilis in pregnancy	Benzathine penicillin G 2.4 MU i.m. single dose (1st and 2nd trimesters) or a second dose after a week in the 3rd trimester (day 8) *or* Procaine penicillin G 600 mg (600 000 units) i.m. once daily for 10 days	Amoxycillin 500 mg orally q.d.s. plus probenacid 500 mg q.d.s. orally for 14 days *or* Ceftriaxone 500 mg i.m. daily for 10 days	
Late syphilis in pregnancy	Manage as non-pregnant but without the use of doxycycline		
Congenital syphilis	Benzathine penicillin sodium 100 000 – 150 000 units/kg daily i.v. (in divided doses) for 10 days *or* Procaine penicillin 50 000 units/kg daily i.m. for 10 days		

Syphilis in pregnancy

- Universal antenatal syphilis screening exists in most countries
- Untreated active syphilis in pregnant women increases the incidence of adverse outcomes of pregnancy almost fivefold
- These include: miscarriage, polyhydramnios, pre-term delivery, hydrops, stillbirth and congenital syphilis
- The risk of vertical transmission depends primarily on the stage of maternal syphilis (and on the stage of pregnancy if a newly acquired infection)
- Vertical transmission is higher in untreated primary or secondary syphilis (60–90%), than early latent syphilis (40%), or late latent syphilis (<10%)
- For treatment regimens in pregnancy, see Table 16.4

Management should be in close liaison with obstetric and paediatric clinicians

Management

General

- The diagnosis and the long-term health implications should be explained in detail and reinforced with clear written information
- Quantitative VDRL/RPR testing (±EIA IgM)should be performed prior to commencing therapy (i.e. on day 1 of treatment) as a baseline for monitoring the response to treatment

Treatment (Table 16.4)

- The aim is to achieve a treponemicidal serum level (and in CSF if neurosyphilis), of antimicrobial
- Penicillin is the first line treatment. A penicillin level of >0.018 mg/L is considered treponemicidal
- Treponemal bacterial division occurs every 33 hours and treatment should cover a number of division times, therefore 7–10 days (early syphilis) or 14–21 days (late syphilis) of treatment is recommended
- Parenteral treatment is preferred as bioavailability is guaranteed however IM injection of benzathine benzylpenicillin is painful so the drug should be reconstituted with 1% lidocaine hydrochloride solution, divided into two equal volumes and administered by deep IM injection into two different sites (e.g. upper outer quadrant of each buttock)
- Desensitization should be considered for individuals with penicillin allergy. Many individuals with a history of penicillin allergy will not display hypersensitivity on re-exposure to penicillin as either they were never allergic to penicillin or the reaction has reduced with time. Expertise is required for skin testing and desensitization
- Although used for treatment of syphilis, both benzathine and procaine penicillin G are unlicensed in the UK (see Chapter 1 for off-label prescribing)

Complications of treatment

Jarisch–Herxheimer reaction

- This is an acute febrile illness associated with the start of antibiotic therapy particularly in early syphilis infection
- Symptoms usually occur within 8 hours and include headache, myalgia and rigours
- The reaction resolves within 24 hours and is not usually clinically significant unless there is neurological or ophthalmogical involvement (severe clinical deterioration in early syphilis with optic neuritis and uveitis has been reported), or if the patient is pregnant (when uterine contractions can occur secondary to fever with a theoretical risk of preterm delivery)
- Patients should be warned of this potential reaction and managed with bed rest and antipyretics. More severe reactions can be treated with corticosteroids
- Steroid cover is recommended when treating cardiovascular syphilis and neurosyphilis (Table 16.4), however there is no evidence that steroids reduce the occurrence of uterine contractions in pregnancy

Procaine reaction

- Also known as Hoignes syndrome, this is a non-allergic reaction to inadvertent intravenous administration of procaine penicillin
- It begins immediately and lasts for less than 20 minutes
- It is characterized by feelings of impeding death and hallucinations and seizures may also occur
- Management is by verbal reassurance, although restraint may be necessary. Rectal diazepam 10 mg should be given if seizures occur. Anaphylaxis should be excluded
- The risk of procaine reaction can be minimized by the aspiration technique of injection

Anaphylaxis

Penicillin is one of the commonest causes of anaphylaxis and facilities for resuscitation must be available.

Partner notification

- Patients with a diagnosis of syphilis should see an appropriate HCP, e.g. a sexual health advisor, with whom PN should be discussed
- Abstinence from any sexual contact should be advised until any lesions (if present) are fully healed and/or after the results of first follow-up serology have been reviewed
- The look-back period for patients with primary syphilis is 3 months. For patients with secondary or early latent syphilis it must extend back to 2 years
- In late syphilis, the index case is not infectious at diagnosis. An estimate of when the infection was acquired should be made and contacts from within 2 years of this time notified. Previous negative serology can be helpful in approximating this
- Asymptomatic contacts of patients with early syphilis should be offered epidemiological treatment in addition to screening, particularly if full surveillance is not possible

Follow-up

- For early syphilis assess (clinically and serologically) at end of treatment and then at 1, 2, 3, 6 and 12 months
- Continue to review 6 monthly until serofast or VDRL/RPR negative
- A four-fold drop in VDRL titre should be expected by 6–12 months (e.g. from 1:32 to 1:8)
- If the VDRL titre shows a fourfold increase at any stage, this is suggestive of treatment failure or reinfection as is the recurrence of signs or symptoms
- If the VDRL/RPR is negative or serofast at 12 months and the patient remains asymptomatic they can be discharged
- It is helpful to provide the patient and their GP with a summary of treatment and discharge serology to prevent unnecessary treatment in the future

17 Genital herpes

Table 17.1 HSV terminology

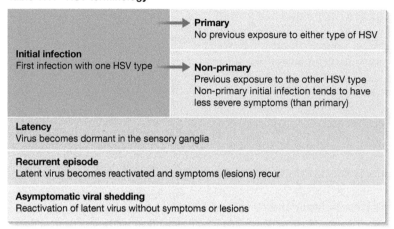

Initial infection First infection with one HSV type	**Primary** No previous exposure to either type of HSV
	Non-primary Previous exposure to the other HSV type Non-primary initial infection tends to have less severe symptoms (than primary)
Latency Virus becomes dormant in the sensory ganglia	
Recurrent episode Latent virus becomes reactivated and symptoms (lesions) recur	
Asymptomatic viral shedding Reactivation of latent virus without symptoms or lesions	

Figure 17.1 Clinical appearance of genital herpes

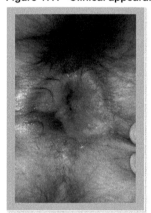

(a) Perianal ulcers
Source: CDC Public Health Image Library

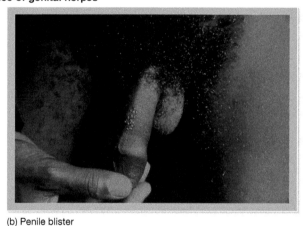

(b) Penile blister
Source: CDC Public Health Image Library/Dr. Paul Wiesner

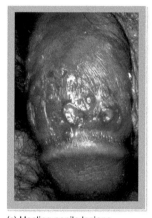

(c) Healing penile lesions
Source: CDC Public Health Image Library
/Dr. N.J. Flumara; Dr. Gavin Hart

Figure 17.2 Herpetic whitlow

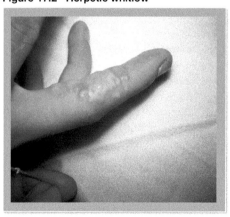

Source: CDC Public Health Image Library/Dr. Thomas Sellers, Emory University

Table 17.2 Recommended antiviral regimens for first episode genital herpes

Immunocompetent individuals		Immunosuppressed individuals (including immunocompromised HIV positive individuals)	
Preferred regimens Aciclovir 400 mg three times daily Valaciclovir 500 mg twice daily	Orally for 5 days	Aciclovir 400 mg five times daily *or*	Orally for 10 days
Alternative regimens Aciclovir 200 mg five times daily Famciclovir 250 mg three times daily*		Valaciclovir 1 g twice daily	

*For episodic management, Famciclovir dose is 125 mg twice daily for 5 days

Sexual and Reproductive Health at a Glance, First Edition. Catriona Melville. © 2015 by John Wiley & Sons, Ltd. Published 2015 by John Wiley & Sons, Ltd.
Companion website: www.ataglanceseries.com/sexualhealth

Background

Genital herpes is a lifelong viral infection characterized by periods of latency and reactivation. Genital herpes infection is caused by the herpes simplex viruses (HSV). There are two types of this DNA virus; HSV-1 and HSV-2. Both can cause genital infection. HSV terminology is explained in Table 17.1.

Aetiology

- HSV-1 is often acquired in childhood manifesting as orolabial herpes (cold sores)
- After childhood, symptomatic primary infection with HSV-1 is equally likely to be acquired in the genital or oral areas
- HSV-2 is traditionally associated with sexual transmission and genital infection
- From adolescence onwards, genital infection with HSV-2 increases in prevalence; however, in the UK the majority of primary and initial genital herpes infections in adults are due to HSV-1
- Most HSV infections are acquired subclinically, with only 30% of individuals developing symptoms at the time of acquisition
- Incubation period is variable but typically 2–14 days
- Transmission is via direct contact with virus which can be shed orally, anorectally, from the external genitalia, cervix or urethra. Transmission is greatest during the viral prodrome (if present) or when there are lesions however asymptomatic shedding probably plays a significant role in onwards transmission of HSV. Condoms are partially effective in preventing genital HSV transmission
- Recurrence: the frequency of recurrences for genital herpes is greater for HSV-2 than HSV-1 (by fourfold). After a symptomatic first episode, the recurrence rate per month for HSV-2 is 0.34 (i.e. approximately 4 recurrences per year). The frequency of recurrences tends to decline over time in most individuals

Clinical features

Symptoms

- Asymptomatic whereby the infection will be unrecognized
- Painful blisters or ulcers
- Dysuria
- Vaginal or urethral discharge
- Systemic symptoms, e.g. myalgia and fever, are commoner in primary HSV (than in initial or recurrent infection)

Signs

- Blisters and ulcers of external genitalia (Figure 17.1) and may involve the cervix and rectum
- Tender inguinal lymphadenitis
- The lesions and lymphadenitis are usually bilateral in first episodes, and unilateral in recurrences (although affected side can alternate)
- Lesions in recurrent episodes may be small and resemble fissures or non-specific erythema. They are limited to the infected dermatome and often affect favoured sites

Diagnosis

The diagnosis should be made from the history, clinical appearance and the following investigations.

Virus detection and typing

- Direct detection of HSV in genital lesions is essential for confirmation of the diagnosis. Typing of the virus (into HSV-1 and HSV-2) aids counselling on prognosis and assists with management of the infection. This is recommended in all patients with first episode genital herpes infection
- Specimens should be collected from the base of an ulcer or from a vesicle. Ideally material from several lesions should be collected to maximize diagnostic yield
- The recommended diagnostic method for HSV detection and virus typing is a NAAT, e.g. PCR, as the detection rates are far superior to HSV culture which was the test traditionally used for diagnosis (HSV culture will miss approximately a third of PCR positive samples)
- PCR tests can tolerate less stringent conditions in terms of storage and transport of specimens
- Swabs from old lesions or from individuals taking antivirals may result in a false-negative result

Herpes serology

- Serological testing for HSV has a limited role in overall herpes management
- Serological testing is not routinely recommended in asymptomatic individuals
- Testing for type-specific antibodies (HSV-1 IgG or HSV-2 IgG or both) can be used for diagnosis, but detection only represents infection with HSV at some point in time (not necessarily recent infection)
- Other HSV antibody tests are generic (not type-specific) and have no value in HSV management
- Serological testing may have a place in managing pregnant women by looking for seroconversion. An early pregnancy serum sample can be compared with a current sample (to demonstrate recent primary infection). It may also be helpful in managing individuals with recurrent genital disease of unknown cause, or for investigating sexual partners of individuals with genital herpes to aid counselling regarding transmission and further management

Dark ground microscopy

- May be appropriate in some clinical situations

Complications

- Urinary retention can occur either due to severe pain or autonomic neuropathy
- Aseptic meningitis
- Superinfection of lesions (e.g. with candida or streptococcal species)
- Autoinoculation to fingers (herpetic Whitlow) (Figure 17.2) and adjacent skin, e.g. thighs

Management

First episode genital herpes

- General measures: saline bathing should be advised and appropriate analgesia prescribed. Topical anaesthetic agents can be of use especially with severe dysuria but occasionally they can cause sensitization, e.g. 5% lidocaine gel. Yellow soft paraffin (Vaseline) can be used on lesions
- Antiviral drugs: patients presenting within 5 days of the start of the episode or while new lesions are still forming should be given oral antiviral drugs (Table 17.2). Aciclovir, valaciclovir and famciclovir all reduce the severity and duration of episodes. The newer antiviral drugs are more expensive than aciclovir with no evidence of additional benefits. If new vesicles are still forming therapy can be extended beyond the initial 5 days. Immunosuppressed individuals are given a longer course with higher drug doses (Table 17.2)

Table 17.3 Episodic treatment, short course regimens

Short course regimens	Comments
Aciclovir 800 mg three times daily for 2 days Famciclovir 1 g twice daily for one day Valaciclovir 500 mg twice daily for 3 days	• No advantage over standard length regimens • A short course with twice-a-day dosing may be simpler and more convenient for patients • Providing there is no evidence of immune failure, standard doses of antivirals should suffice in people with HIV

Table 17.4 Suppressive treatment regimens

Aciclovir 400 mg twice daily Aciclovir 200 mg four times daily Famciclovir 250 mg twice daily Valaciclovir 500 mg daily	Suppressive therapy should be provided for a minimum of 6 months and discontinued after 12 months of continuous treatment to reassess recurrence frequency

Figure 17.3 Genital herpes in pregnancy

Primary HSV	Both primary and recurrent HSV infection carry a risk of neonatal herpes infection	Recurrent HSV (initial episode predates pregnancy)

Primary HSV

1st and 2nd trimester acquisition

• Aciclovir is not licensed for use in pregnancy however is considered safe and is not associated with birth defects

• Manage episode in line with clinical condition and anticipate vaginal delivery

• Consider suppressive aciclovir therapy from 36 weeks' gestation

3rd trimester

• Associated with most risk as viral shedding may persist and delivery may occur before development of protective maternal antibodies

• 41% risk of neonatal herpes if primary episode HSV lesions are present at time of (vaginal) delivery

• May be associated with preterm labour and low birth weight (although conflicting data)

• Caesarean section should be recommended to all women presenting with primary HSV lesions at or within 6 weeks of delivery

• Type-specific HSV serology is advised to distinguish a primary episode from recurrent infection. If serology demonstrates the same type of HSV isolated from genital swabs then this episode is a recurrence and should be managed as such

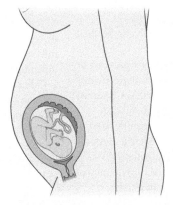

Suppressive therapy
400 mg aciclovir t.d.s. orally

Recurrent HSV (initial episode predates pregnancy)

• Antiviral treatment is rarely indicated

• The risk of neonatal herpes is low (up to 3% when lesions present at delivery)

• Maternal antibodies (IgG) have a protective effect

• Episodes are likely to be brief

• Aciclovir suppressive treatment can be considered from 36 weeks' gestation

• An episode during the antenatal period is not an indication for caesarean section

• If no lesions are present at delivery, vaginal delivery is appropriate

• Caesarean section is not routinely recommended if lesions are present at onset of labour

Table 17.5 Preventing HSV acquisition in pregnancy

Women should be asked at their booking visit if they have a history of genital herpes
Female partners of men with genital herpes who have no history of infection themselves should be advised how to minimise the risk of acquiring the infection in pregnancy by: • Using condoms consistently and correctly especially in the 3rd trimester • Abstaining from sexual intercourse when lesions are present and in the last 6 weeks of pregnancy • Avoiding receptive orogenital contact if her partner has orolabial lesions ('cold-sores')
All women should undergo careful inspection of the vulva at the onset of labour
Women, staff and others in contact with the neonate who have active oral HSV lesions should avoid direct contact between the lesions and the neonate, i.e. by practicing good hand hygiene and not kissing the neonate

Table 17.6 Neonatal herpes

UK incidence 1.65 - 17.5 per 100 000 live births
3 subtypes of disease: • Localized to skin, eyes or mouth • Encephalitis/CNS disease • Disseminated infection (carries the highest mortality ~30%)
> 90% cases are due to direct contact with infected maternal secretions at the time of delivery
Postnatal transmission can occur but is uncommon
Congenital HSV is due to transplacental intrauterine infection and is rare

- Management of complications: admission to hospital may be required for urinary retention, meningism or severe pain/systemic symptoms

Recurrent genital herpes

Recurrent episodes are usually self-limiting and associated with minor symptoms. There are three main management strategies for recurrences.

Supportive therapy

- Suitable for individuals with short, infrequent recurrences which cause minimal discomfort
- As with first episodes, analgesia, saline bathing and the use of soft yellow paraffin are recommended

Episodic antiviral therapy

- Suitable for individuals with infrequent recurrences which are severe and/or long lasting. It can also be useful to provide antiviral cover for a specific occasion, e.g. a holiday. Prompt treatment is necessary and therefore providing advance supplies for patient initiated treatment should be considered
- Treatment with oral aciclovir, valaciclovir or famciclovir reduces the duration of recurrent genital herpes by a median of 1–2 days. The severity of the recurrence is also reduced
- Treatment initiated prior to the development of papules confers the most benefit. Aborted lesions have been documented in up to 30% of individuals with early treatment
- A standard (Table 17.2) or short course (Table 17.3) of treatment can be given. Both are equally effective

Suppressive antiviral therapy (Table 17.4)

- Individuals with a recurrence rate of more than six episodes of genital herpes each year are likely to experience a substantial reduction in recurrence frequency with suppressive therapy
- Individuals with lower rates of recurrences will probably also have fewer recurrences with this regimen
- Before embarking on suppressive therapy consideration should be given to the advantages and disadvantages of treatment including inconvenience and cost
- Suppressive therapy may benefit individuals who have significant associated psychological morbidity from their diagnosis
- Safety and resistance data is most extensive with aciclovir. There is no evidence that valaciclovir or famciclovir offer any clinical advantages and are more expensive than aciclovir so in many services it is the drug of choice (Table 17.4)
- Suppressive therapy with aciclovir requires no monitoring in healthy individuals however the dose should be adjusted in individuals with severe renal disease
- The optimal daily dose of aciclovir is 800 mg. Twice daily dosage seems to be marginally less effective than taking the drug four times a day, but this must be balanced with the ability to adhere to this regimen
- Most individuals will have an episode soon after stopping suppressive therapy. The trial of discontinuation after 12 months should encompass two recurrences. If the frequency and severity of recurrences remains unacceptable it is safe to restart treatment

Asymptomatic viral shedding

This occurs with both types of HSV and is reduced by all antiviral therapies (by 80–90%). It is an important cause of onward transmission of the virus. In some individuals the number of days of asymptomatic shedding exceeds the number of days of symptomatic shedding.

Reducing transmission

- Abstinence should be advised during symptomatic recurrences (including during the prodrome)
- Male condoms may be partially effective in reducing transmission of HSV if used consistently and correctly. The protective effect is greater for women (from acquisition from a male partner)
- Educating patients to recognize the symptoms of recurrences can play a role in preventing transmission
- Aciclovir, famciclovir and valaciclovir suppress symptomatic and asymptomatic viral shedding

Partner notification

Involving the current sexual partner(s) in the counselling process can help relieve anxiety about the diagnosis and support the individual. Confirmation of HSV status in the partner can aid management; however, given the limitations of serology and the non-specific features of genital herpes infection this is not always possible. The legal requirement for disclosure of the diagnosis in relationships is unclear however this issue should be raised with the index patient (and documented by the clinician) as it may offer protection against future legal proceedings.

Support and counselling

Patients with genital herpes can be extremely distressed by the diagnosis and referral to a sexual health advisor is important to provide the necessary support and information about the condition. Counselling should include information giving about the natural history of the infection; subclinical shedding; the risks of transmission; condom use and issues relating to infection in pregnancy. Antiviral treatment can assist adjustment to the diagnosis and reduce anxiety. Information should be provided in writing as well as verbally an should include contact details for local or national support groups, e.g. the Herpes Viruses Association www.herpes.org.uk

Herpes in pregnancy (Figure 17.3, Table 17.5)

- All individuals presenting with genital HSV in pregnancy should be seen by a senior clinician and have their care managed in conjunction with the obstetric and neonatal team
- The incidence of neonatal herpes (Table 17.6) has increased in the UK and has a high morbidity and mortality. The risks of transmission to the neonate are greatest when a new infection occurs in the third trimester

HIV infection and immunodeficiency

- HSV activates HIV replication and may facilitate onward transmission of HIV
- HSV infection increases the chance of HIV acquisition
- Genital herpes is the commonest STI in HIV-positive heterosexuals in the UK
- The degree of HIV associated immunosuppression dictates the likelihood of HSV reactivation. HAART reduces the frequency of clinical recurrences
- Primary HSV in untreated HIV infected individuals can be severe and prolonged with the risk of progression to serious systemic complications, e.g. neurological disease, pneumonia
- Antiviral drug doses are higher in the primary episode and given for longer (Table 17.2)
- Resistance to aciclovir is more common in individuals with HIV co-infection (found in around 5–7% isolates in this group)

18 Genital ulcers: tropical infections

Table 18.1 Differential diagnosis of genital ulcers

STI ætiologies	Anogenital herpes (HSV) Syphilis Chancroid Lymphogranuloma venereum (LGV) Granuloma inguinale (donovanosis)
Non-STI ætiologies	Trauma Fixed drug eruptions and allergy Herpes zoster Cutaneous tuberculosis Behçet's disease (rare) Malignancy Inflammatory bowel disease

Figure 18.1 Clinical appearance of chancroid

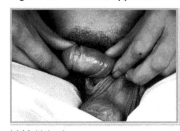
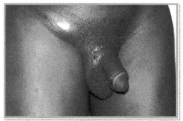

(a) Multiple ulcers
Source: CDC Public Health Image Library/
Dr. Pirozzi

(b) Unilateral bubo and penile ulcer
Source: CDC Public Health Image Library/
J. Pledger

Table 18.2 Clinical features of STI causes of genital ulcers

	Organism	Primary lesion	Number of lesions	Appearance	Pain	Lymphadenopathy
HSV	Herpes simplex virus	Vesicle	Multiple	Superficial, non-indurated	Usually painful	Tender, bilateral
Syphilis	*Treponema pallidum*	Papule	Usually solitary	Well-demarcated ulcer (chancre) with a clean base and indurated border	Usually painless	Non-tender, unilateral, firm
Chancroid	*Haemophilus ducreyi*	Pustule	Multiple	Non-indurated (soft), with ragged border and friable base; covered with a necrotic, often purulent exudate	Usually painful	Very tender (may suppurate - buboes)
LGV	*Chlamydia trachomatis* L1,2,3	Papule	Usually solitary	Small, shallow, transient ulcer, no induration	Usually painless (variable)	Tender, unilateral 'groove sign'
Donovanosis	*Klebsiella granulomatis*	Papule	Variable	Beefy red (vascular) ulcers	Uncommon	Uncommon 'pseudobuboe'

Table 18.3 Recommended treatment regimens for chancroid

Drug regimen	Comments
Azithromycin 1 g orally single dose *or*	Single dose regimens are useful for compliance
Ceftriaxone 250 mg i.m. single dose *or*	
Ciprofloxacin 500 mg orally b.d. for three days *or*	Contraindicated in pregnancy and breastfeeding
Erythromycin 500 mg orally four times a day for 7 days	This is the first line regimen recommended by WHO, however it can cause gastrointestinal upset and compliance may be an issue. It is recommended for HIV positive patients and also for those with allergy to cephalosporins or quinolones

Sexual and Reproductive Health at a Glance, First Edition. Catriona Melville. © 2015 by John Wiley & Sons, Ltd. Published 2015 by John Wiley & Sons, Ltd.
Companion website: www.ataglanceseries.com/sexualhealth

Background

Genital ulcers are breaches in the skin or mucous membranes. They can occur anywhere in the anogenital region.

They can be caused by infectious or non-infectious aetiologies (Table 18.1). In industrialized countries, genital ulcer disease (GUD) due to STIs is most likely to be herpetic (HSV) in origin. Infection with several different organisms can occur in the same individual. Clinical features of sexually transmitted genital ulcer infections are summarized in Table 18.2.

Chancroid

Aetiology and epidemiology

- Caused by the organism *Haemophilus ducreyi* a small anaerobic Gram-negative coccobacillus
- Although still endemic in regions of some countries (e.g. Africa, Asia), the prevalence has declined markedly in many developing countries. The reasons for this decline include; increased condom use in high-risk groups, the introduction of more effective antibiotics for GUD and identifying and managing chancroid as a means of controlling the spread of HIV
- Chancroid is rare in modernized countries although discrete outbreaks can occur, often in association with sex workers
- *Incubation period*: 3–7 days
- *Transmission*: sexually transmitted including orogenital contact. No evidence of congenital or perinatal transmission. Local auto-inoculation can occur by fingers. Male circumcision is highly protective against infection. Chancroid is a major cofactor in the heterosexual transmission of HIV

Symptoms and signs

- No prodromal symptoms
- A tender red papule develops into a pustule and then progresses to single or multiple painful ulcers or soft (non-indurated) sores (Figure 18.1)
- Ulcers are usually 1–2 cm in diameter, have a ragged edge and a yellow or grey base which bleeds on contact
- Sites of infection:
  - Men: prepuce, coronal sulcus, frenulum, glans penis
  - Women: vulva especially labia minora and fourchette. Vaginal and cervical lesions are uncommon
  - Extragenital lesions: extremely uncommon, fingers, breasts and inner thighs
- Inguinal lymphadenopathy: usually unilateral and painful, occurs in 50% of cases in men but less often in women. This presents as a tender inguinal swelling which can develop into a unilocular abscess (a bubo). Buboes usually appear 7–10 days after the initial lesion
- Clinical variants: lesions can coalesce into giant phagadenic ulcers; they can be small and look similar to herpes, or they can be solitary and painless mimicking syphilis
- There is no systemic dissemination of infection
- *H. ducreyi* can be carried asymptomatically. This has been reported in sex workers and is an important reservoir of infection

Complications

Bacterial superinfection with tissue destruction; phimosis following infection of the prepuce; chronic suppurative inguinal sinuses.

Diagnosis

Investigations

- *H. ducreyi* is a fastidious organism requiring blood enriched medium for culture. A sample can be taken from the ulcer base after removing superficial pus, and directly plated onto culture medium. The culture plate must be incubated for a minimum of 48–72 hours in high humidity at 33° with 5% carbon dioxide
- PCR tests to detect *H. ducreyi* DNA are under development, although in most countries commercial assays are not yet available and PCR can only be performed at research or specialized laboratories
- Microscopy of a Gram-stained smear of material from the cleaned ulcer may show chains of small Gram-negative coccobacilli. The sensitivity of Gram-stain is only 50%
- Where available, PCR is the most sensitive technique (sensitivity >95%), followed by culture (sensitivity <80%)

Presumptive diagnosis

As direct detection of *H. Ducreyi* can be problematic, a presumptive diagnosis can be made if the clinical presentation is characteristic for chancroid, e.g. painful genital ulceration and regional lymphadenopathy with negative tests for syphilis and herpes.

Management

General: Advise abstinence from sexual intercourse until treatment is completed for both the individual and their partner(s), screen for other causes of GUD and STIs, and give information about the condition.

Treatment: recommended antibiotics are listed in Table 18.3. Fluctuant buboes should be aspirated by needle with antibiotic cover.

Follow-up: review should occur 3–7 days after initiation of therapy. Clinical improvement should occur within this timescale. Large ulcers and buboes may take longer to heal, e.g. ≥2 weeks.

Test of cure: not recommended.

Partner notification: the 'look back' period for chancroid is 10 days. Sexual contacts should be examined and treated even if they have no symptoms. Screening is not recommended.

Lymphogranuloma venereum (LGV)

Aetiology and epidemiology

- An STI caused by L1, L2 (most commonly) or L3 serovars of *Chlamydia trachomatis* (Table 10.1)
- Prior to 2003 LGV was viewed mainly as a tropical disease. It was rarely seen in industrialized countries and usually only in individuals who had travelled to endemic regions e.g. Southern and West Africa, South-East Asia, India, Madagascar and the Caribbean
- Since 2003 a series of outbreaks have occurred across Europe and other developed countries mainly in HIV-positive MSM
- The UK has had the highest number of cases globally since 2004. These are often associated with the sex party scene in London, Brighton and Manchester; 99% of cases are in MSM of which approximately 80% are HIV positive

Figure 18.2   The groove sign in LGV

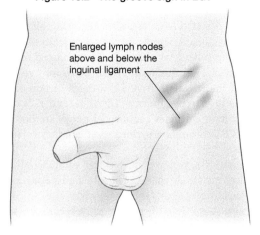

Enlarged lymph nodes above and below the inguinal ligament

Figure 18.3   Lesions in *Donovanosis*

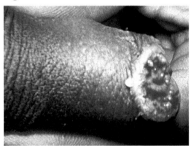

Source: CDC Public Health Image Library/Joyce Ayers

Table 18.5 Recommended treatment regimens for *Donovanosis*

Drug regimen
Azithromycin 1 g weekly *or* 500 mg daily orally Doxycycline 100 mg b.d. orally Erythromycin 500 mg q.i.d. orally

Notes

- Duration of all treatments is until lesions have healed or a minimum of 3 weeks
- In pregnancy and breastfeeding, erythromycin should be used

Table 18.4   Recommended treatment regimens for LGV

Drug regimen	Comments
Doxycycline 100 mg b.d. orally for 21 days	Recommended first-line treatment
Erythromycin 500 mg q.i.d. orally for 21 days	Use in pregnancy, breastfeeding or tetracycline allergy

Figure 18.4   Giemsa-stained smear showing Donovan bodies

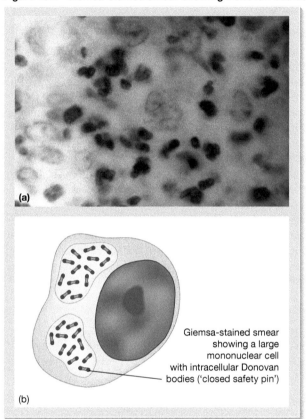

(a)

(b)

Giemsa-stained smear showing a large mononuclear cell with intracellular Donovan bodies ('closed safety pin')

Source: CDC Public Health Image Library/Susan Lindsley

- The small number of cases in heterosexuals appear to be linked to bisexual male partners or overseas travel
- *Incubation period*: 3–30 days
- *Transmission*: sexually transmitted including orogenital and anal contact. No evidence of congenital infection but LGV may be acquired perinatally from the birth canal

Clinical features

Divided into three stages:

Primary LGV

- Small painless papule, pustule or shallow ulcer. Often unnoticed. Sites include the coronal sulcus and glans penis in men and in women the posterior vaginal wall, fourchette , vulva or cervix (rare). Extra-genital lesions can be oral (lip or tonsils) or perianal (MSM)
- LGV proctitis in MSM: symptoms include; anorectal bleeding, rectal pain, rectal discharge, constipation or tenesmus. Almost all recent cases in MSM in Western Europe have presented with haemorrhagic proctitis. A small number have presented with 'classical' genital lesions. Rectal LGV can be asymptomatic
- LGV pharyngitis has been reported in MSM

Secondary LGV (inguinal syndrome)

- Regional dissemination causes tender lymphadenopathy usually 1–6 weeks after the primary lesion
- Usually presents as tender, unilateral (in 2/3) inguinal and/or femoral lymphadenopathy. This can progress to bubo formation. Chronic fistulae can occur as a result of ruptured buboes
- The 'groove' sign occurs in 15–20% of cases (Figure 18.2)
- Dissemination may be associated with systemic symptoms namely fever, arthritis, pneumonitis and rarely perihepatitis with deranged liver enzymes
- Most patients recover at this stage

Tertiary LGV (genito-anorectal syndrome)

- In a minority of patients infection will persist in the anogenital tissues causing chronic inflammation and tissue destruction which can mimic Crohn's disease (e.g. proctitis, proctocolitis, strictures and fistulae). Fibrosis and scarring of the vulva can occur with esthiomene (from the Greek word meaning 'eaten away')
- Occurs most commonly in women due to the retroperitoneal lymphatic drainage of the vulva and vagina

Complications

- Genital lymphoedema due to lymph node destruction
- There is a reported association with rectal carcinoma

Diagnosis

There should be a high index of clinical suspicion especially in MSM with rectal symptoms. Testing for alternative and co-existing pathologies should be undertaken.

Investigations

- NAAT testing for LGV-specific DNA (e.g. PCR) is available at reference laboratories in the UK and other developed countries
- Samples can be collected from the ulcer base, or swabs taken from the rectum, pharynx or urethra
- Culture has a much lower sensitivity than PCR and is not readily available. *Chlamydia* serology is only performed in a few specialized laboratories
- Biopsy of lesions or lymph nodes for histology may be required to differentiate LGV from other pathologies

- A full sexual health screen should be offered including testing for other causes of GUD (and/or proctitis), e.g. syphilis, HSV and gonorrohoea. Given the high incidence of co-infection with HIV and HCV, testing for these infections is recommended

Management

General: Advise abstinence from sexual intercourse until treatment is completed for both the individual and their partner(s). Detailed information about the condition should be given.
Treatment: Recommended antibiotics are listed in Table 18.4.
Follow-up: signs and symptoms usually resolve within 1–2 weeks for early infection. Review should include confirmation of adequate PN and repeat BBV testing if applicable.
Test of cure: not recommended if course of treatment completed with the exception of infection in pregnancy. If indicated defer NAAT testing until 2 weeks after antibiotics completed.
Partner notification: the 'look back' period is 4 weeks for symptomatic LGV and 3 months for asymptomatic infection. Sexual contacts should be examined, tested and treated.

Donovanosis (granuloma inguinale)

Aetiology and epidemiology

- Caused by the Gram-negative bacterium *Klebsiella granulomatis*
- Small endemic foci in tropical and sub-tropical countries, e.g. Papua New Guinea, India, Vietnam, the Caribbean and also in Indigenous Australians (central and northern Australia)
- *Incubation period*: uncertain but likely to be 40–50 days (up to 6 months)
- *Transmission*: direct sexual contact; rarely through non-sexual skin contact

Symptoms and signs (Figure 18.3)

- One or more papules/nodules develop at site of primary inoculation (genital, anal, oral). These progress to (usually) painless, friable ulcers which increase in size
- Untreated infections may heal spontaneously or become necrotic and spread locally with tissue destruction
- Lymphadenopathy uncommon unless secondary bacterial infection. Pseudobuboes may occur (subcutaneous granulomatous nodules which can mimic buboes)

Complications

- Genital lymphoedema (elephantitis), squamous carcinoma and rarely haematogenous dissemination to bone and viscera

Diagnosis

- Demonstration of intracellular Donovan bodies either from a tissues sample (lesion biopsy) or cellular material from a swab stained with Giemsa stain (Figure 18.4)
- Donovan bodies appear as Gram-negative bacteria often with bipolar inclusions producing a safety pin appearance
- Cell culture and PCR described but not readily available

Management

Treatment: recommended antibiotics are listed in Table 18.5.
Follow-up: until symptoms have resolved.
Partner notification: look-back period for PN is 40 days before the onset of lesions. Sexual contacts should be assessed and offered treatment.

19 Epididymo-orchitis and sexually-acquired reactive arthritis

Figure 19.1 Differential diagnosis of epididymo-orchitis

- STIs e.g. *Chlamydia trachomatis, Neisseria gonorrhoeae*
- Non-STI Gram-negative enteric organisms (complication of UTI)
- Testicular torsion
- Testicular tumour
- Mumps (orchitis occurs in up to 30% post-pubertal infected men)
- Amiodarone (drug side-effect)
- Behçet's disease (occurs in up to 19%) ⎤
- Extrapulmonary tuberculosis   ⎬ — Rare
- Other infections: *Candida, Brucella*   ⎦

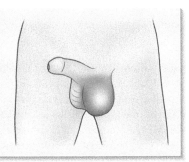

Table 19.1 Treatment for epididymo-orchitis

Most likely any STI pathogen	Ceftriaxone 500 mg i.m. single dose plus Doxycycline 100 mg orally b.d. for 14 days
Most likely non-gonococcal STI (i.e negative microscopy, low risk group)	Doxycycline 100 mg orally b.d. for 14 days *or* Ofloxacin 200 mg orally b.d. 14 days
Most likely enteric organisms	Ciprofloxacin 500 mg orally b.d. 10 days *or* Ofloxacin 200 mg orally b.d. 14 days

Box 19.1 Testicular torsion (torsion of the spermatic cord)

- Surgical emergency: treatment is required within 6 hours to avoid irreversible ischaemic injury
- More common in men < 20 years
- Often acute onset of severe unilateral pain
- Testis may lie transversely or high in the scrotum
- Doppler ultrasound of the scrotum to assess presence of testicular blood flow (sensitivity not 100% therefore do not delay surgical exploration of the scrotum if indicated)

Figure 19.2 Clinical features of SARA

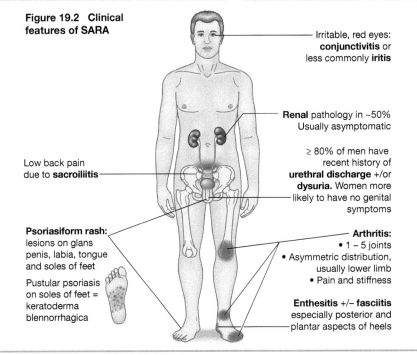

Irritable, red eyes: **conjunctivitis** or less commonly **iritis**

Renal pathology in ~50% Usually asymptomatic

≥ 80% of men have recent history of **urethral discharge** +/or **dysuria**. Women more likely to have no genital symptoms

Low back pain due to **sacroiliitis**

Psoriasiform rash: lesions on glans penis, labia, tongue and soles of feet

Pustular psoriasis on soles of feet = keratoderma blennorrhagica

Arthritis:
- 1 – 5 joints
- Asymmetric distribution, usually lower limb
- Pain and stiffness

Enthesitis +/− fasciitis especially posterior and plantar aspects of heels

Sexual and Reproductive Health at a Glance, First Edition. Catriona Melville. © 2015 by John Wiley & Sons, Ltd. Published 2015 by John Wiley & Sons, Ltd.
Companion website: www.ataglanceseries.com/sexualhealth

Epididymo-orchitis

Definition: inflammation, pain and swelling of the epididymis (epididymitis), testes (orchitis) or both.

Aetiology: Usually due to local spread of infection from the urethra (STI) or the bladder (urinary tract infection – UTI). Causes are listed in Figure 19.1. Under aged 35 years it is most commonly caused by a sexually transmitted pathogen. Over aged 35 years it is more likely to be a complication of a UTI (i.e. Gram-negative enteric organisms). Enteric organisms can also be transmitted sexually in men who have insertive anal intercourse. The most important diagnosis to exclude in all men is testicular torsion (Box 19.1). If there is suspicion of a testicular tumour an urgent referral should be made. There has been a recent resurgence of mumps in the UK, especially in non-vaccinated adults.

Symptoms: (usually) unilateral pain and swelling. Urethral discharge ± dysuria (if due to an STI); symptoms of UTI (frequency, pyrexia); headache, fever and parotid swelling may precede unilateral testicular swelling in mumps by 7–10 days, although one third of patients with mumps do not develop parotitis.

Signs: scrotal erythema and oedema, tenderness to palpation, epididymal swelling, urethral discharge, secondary hydrocoele, pyrexia.

Complications: hydrocoele, abscess and testicular infarction (rare), infertility or subfertility, testicular atrophy (post-mumps) causes reduced fertility in 13% men with bilateral disease.

Diagnosis and investigations: Testicular torsion should be excluded first and referral expedited if any suspicion of this diagnosis. Always exclude STIs; NAAT for *C. trachomatis* and *N. gonorrhoeae*; Gram-stained urethral smear if available may show urethritis ± Gram-negative intracellular diplococci; urine dipstick for nitrites, leucocytes and blood (UTI); microscopy and culture of mid-stream urine specimen. All men with a confirmed UTI should be referred for further assessment of the urinary tract. Three early morning urines should be sent if suspicion of TB (also CXR etc.). Mumps is diagnosed by IgM/IgG serology.

Management

General: rest, scrotal support, analgesia (including NSAIDs). Advise abstinence from SI until they and their partners have completed treatment and follow-up if a sexually transmitted cause is suspected or confirmed. Give written information on the condition.

Treatment: empirical antibiotic treatment should be given to all patients (before results are available). The chosen regimen should be in accordance with local antibiotic sensitivities (Table 19.1). Inpatient hospital treatment should be considered in individuals with features of bacteraemia or severe disease.

PN: all current partners should be tested and offered epidemiological treatment unless a non-STI cause is confirmed.

Follow-up: Diagnosis should be reviewed if no improvement in 3 days, or symptoms worsen. Reassess again at 2 weeks to confirm compliance with therapy, PN, and clinical improvement. TOC is required for gonorrhoea (see Chapter 11).

Sexually acquired reactive arthritis (SARA)

Definition: reactive arthritis (ReA) is a seronegative, inflammation of the synovial membrane initiated by an infection at a distant site. If the trigger is an STI then it is referred to as SARA. This includes Reiter's syndrome (triad of conjunctivitis, urethritis and arthritis).

Aetiology: Most frequently associated with chlamydia infection (35–69% of cases), and also linked with *Neisseria gonorrhoeae* and *Ureaplasma urealyticum*. Occurs ten times more frequently in men than in women (although under diagnosis in women may occur).

Pathogenesis: appears to involve an immune response to urogenital microorganisms. There may be a personal or family history of spondyloarthritis. Susceptibility is markedly increased by possession of the HLA-B27 gene.

Symptoms and signs (Figure 19.2): usually start within 30 days of SI. 10% will also have systemic symptoms of malaise, fever and fatigue. Urethritis, cervicitis, epidiymitis, tenosynovitis with crepitus (especially fingers) and circinate balanitis may manifest.

Complications: SARA is self-limiting in the majority of individuals. The mean duration of the first episode is 4–6 months. 50% of individuals will have recurrent episodes. Complications are primarily due to aggressive arthritis and are more frequent in those who are HLA-B27 positive. Erosive damage to joints causes locomotor disability in 15%. Complications of anterior uveitis include cataract formation and blindness.

Diagnosis: clinical. Enquire about joint, eye and skin symptoms in patients with urethral symptoms. Ask about new sexual partners and symptoms of STIs in individuals with symptoms of SARA.

Investigations: full STI screen, ESR, FBC or CRP and urinalysis are essential tests. LFTs, and renal function tests and X-rays of affected joints may be useful depending on the clinical picture. Exclusion tests for other causes of arthritis may be indicated, e.g. plasma urate for gout.

Management

General: Rest and NSAIDs. Advise abstinence from SI including oral sex until treatment and PN completed.

Treatment: Standard antibiotic regimens for specific diagnosed genital infections (see relevant chapters). The role of longer courses of antibiotics is contentious. Ideally manage the individual in conjunction with rheumatology/ophthalmology/dermatology. Arthritis should be treated with rest, physiotherapy and regular NSAIDs (assess gastrointestinal haemorrhage risk). Intra-articular corticosteroid injections may be helpful for single joints. Second line therapies should be commenced in liaison with a rheumatologist.

PN: the look back period depends on the genital infection diagnosed (see relevant chapters).

Follow-up: as per STI diagnosed. Specialists should determine follow-up for extra-genital manifestations.

Acute bacterial prostatitis

A rare, but potentially serious bacterial infection caused by urinary pathogens, e.g. *Escherichia coli*, enterococci. Suspect in men presenting with urinary voiding symptoms and systemic symptoms (e.g. fever, myalgia, rigors). Treat with antibiotics and analgesia while awaiting results of urine culture, e.g. ciprofloxacin 500 mg p.o. b.d. for 28 days.

Molluscum contagiosum and normal genital lumps

Figure 20.1 Molluscum contagiosum

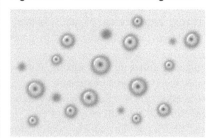

Box 20.1 Differential diagnosis of molluscum contagiosum

- Physiological /normal genital skin
- Anogenital warts
- Ectopic sebaceous glands
- Keratoacanthoma
- Basal cell carcinoma
- Dermatofibroma
- Disseminated fungal infections in late immunosuppression, e.g. cryptococcosis, aspergillosis

Figure 20.3 Normal anatomical variations of vulva and cervix

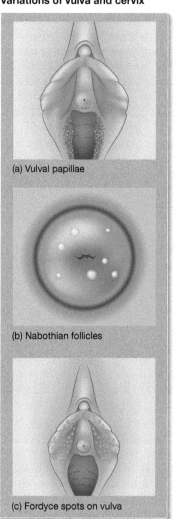

(a) Vulval papillae

(b) Nabothian follicles

(c) Fordyce spots on vulva

Figure 20.2 Molluscum contagiosum infection in immunocompromised individuals

Causes
Malignancy, immunosuppressant treatments, late HIV infection

Signs
Larger and more severe infection often with ≥ 100 lesions

Location
Lesions commonly affect the face and neck, especially eyelids

Complications
Can cause a foreign body type reaction → chronic conjunctivitis

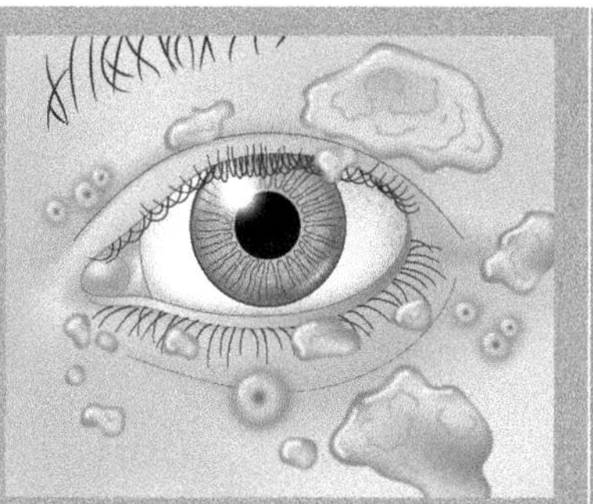

Figure 20.4 Normal anatomical variations of the penis

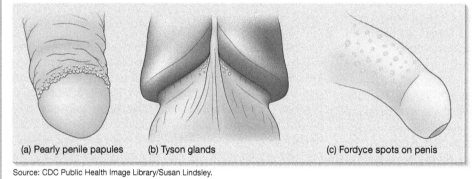

(a) Pearly penile papules   (b) Tyson glands   (c) Fordyce spots on penis

Source: CDC Public Health Image Library/Susan Lindsley.

Sexual and Reproductive Health at a Glance, First Edition. Catriona Melville. © 2015 by John Wiley & Sons, Ltd. Published 2015 by John Wiley & Sons, Ltd.
Companion website: www.ataglanceseries.com/sexualhealth

Molluscum contagiosum

Genital molluscum is a common benign, self-limiting skin condition caused by the Molluscum contagiosum virus (MCV). MCV is a large DNA type of Pox virus from the *Molluscipox* genus.

Aetiology

- Molluscum infection can occur in adults and children
- The vast majority of infections are seen in children and infants where it usually affects the trunk, face and neck or limbs and is non-sexually transmitted
- Genital infection in adults is usually acquired through sexual contact with lesions affecting the genitals, pubic region, lower abdomen, buttocks and upper thighs
- It affects males and females in equal proportions
- *Transmission*: direct skin to skin contact or autoinoculation through excoriation of lesions. Transmission occasionally occurs via fomites (e.g. shared towels). It is not transmitted vertically or perinatally
- *Incubation period*: 1 week to 6 months
- Facial lesions are associated with HIV infection
- Severe infection with large lesions can occur with HIV associated immunodeficiency
- *Natural history*: the infection is self-limiting in immunocompetent individuals. Lesions will regress spontaneously over several (3–9) months

Symptoms

Individuals commonly present complaining of genital lumps which they may have self-diagnosed (incorrectly) as genital warts. Otherwise molluscum are generally symptomless although they can be associated with itch.

Signs

- Lesions are discrete, pearly and smooth and often have an umbilicated centre (Figure 20.1)
- They are usually 2–5 mm in diameter and can occur individually or in clusters
- Infection is associated with up to 30 lesions at a time unless immunosuppressed
- Lesions can occur anywhere on the body
- An inflammatory dermatitis can develop around the lesions and there may be signs of secondary bacterial infection. As they resolve, they appear inflamed or crusty

Diagnosis

The diagnosis is made clinically by the characteristic appearance. The differential diagnosis is listed in (Box 20.1). There is no need for laboratory confirmation.

Complications

- Secondary bacterial infections can occur if lesions are scratched
- Up to a third of individuals will have recurrences over the subsequent 1–2 years
- Infection in immunocompromised individuals (Figure 20.2)

Management

General

- Offer STI testing if appropriate and in particular HIV testing in individuals with facial lesions
- Advice about autoinoculation should be given. The central plug of the molluscum lesion contains infectious virus and squeezing them can easily spread the infection
- Towels and bed-linen should not be shared when active lesions are present

Treatment

- Treatment is for cosmetic reasons only therefore an expectant approach is a suitable option in view of the natural history of the virus
- Lesions can be treated with cryotherapy (liquid nitrogen) and repeated at weekly intervals. This is also suitable for pregnant women
- Second line treatments include Podophyllotoxin cream (0.5%) or Imiquimod cream (5%). They are both unlicensed for this indication and are contraindicated in pregnancy and breastfeeding. The regimens are the same as for anogenital warts
- Other: curettage is suitable for non-genital and non-facial lesions but is painful; various chemical preparations, e.g. phenol can be used but these lack supporting evidence particularly for use in the genital area. Individual lesions can be pierced and the core manually expressed although care must be taken not to spread the virus or cause secondary infection
- In patients with immunodeficiency due to HIV infection, anti-retroviral therapy may assist in resolution of lesions

Follow-up and partner issues

No follow-up or partner notification is required unless another STI is diagnosed.

Physiological genital lumps

Normal/physiological genital lumps or anatomical variations are common in both men and women and can cause unnecessary anxiety if they are mistaken for an STI or a pathological anogenital lesion. Reassurance regarding normal anatomy is essential. Treatment is not indicated for any of the following variations of normal anatomy (Figures 20.3 and 20.4).

- Fordyce spots: ectopic sebaceous glands, 2–5 mm, pale, smooth and soft, often found on the prepuce in males and upper inner labia minora in females
- Pearly penile papules (hirsutes papillaris penis): one to three rows of smooth, discrete, white, dome-shaped, non-coalescing papules, 1–2 mm in size, edging the corona of the penis and adjacent to the frenum. Often mistaken for genital warts. Present in up to 50% of men. Do not require treatment
- Vulval papillae: small, soft, pink, frond-like fleshy papules commonly found within the labia minora and vestibule. They are largely symmetrical and can be mistaken for genital warts
- Tyson's glands: 1–2 mm regular paired glands, on either side of the penile frenulum just proximal to the coronal sulcus
- Nabothian follicles: physiological cervical retention cysts. Appear as bluish or yellow translucent lumps on the ectocervix
- Foreskin remnants (in circumcised men) or hymenal remnants in women
- Angiokeratomas: deep red or purple papules usually over the scrotum but can also appear on the shaft of the penis and labia majora, due to benign hyperkeratosis with dilated capillaries
- Acrochordons (skin tags):commonly in the over 50s, around the groin and thighs

21 Anogenital warts and human papilloma virus infection

Table 21.1 Predominant types of HPV found in different lesions

Manifestation	HPV type	
Common skin warts	1, 2, 3, 4, 26, 27	
Anogenital warts	6, 11	Cause > 90% of genital warts, but co-infection with multiple strains can occur
Laryngeal papilloma	6, 11	
Cervical squamous cell carcinoma	16, 18	Cause ~70% cervical cancers
Oropharyngeal carcinoma	16	
Anogenital squamous intraepithelial lesions i.e. AIN, CIN, PIN, VIN, VAIN*	16, 18	

*Anal, cervical, penile, vulval, and vaginal intraepithelial neoplasia

Box 21.1 Differential diagnosis of anogenital warts

→ Normal anatomy, e.g. pearly penile papules, Fordyce spots, nabothian follicles (cervix), vulval papillae
→ Skin tags
→ Molluscum contagiosum
→ Condyloma lata (2ry syphilis)
→ Epidermoid cysts
→ Dermatofibromas
→ Intra-epithelial neoplasia
→ Malignant lesions

Figure 21.1 Genital warts on (a) penis and (b) perianal region

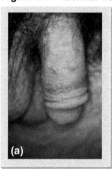 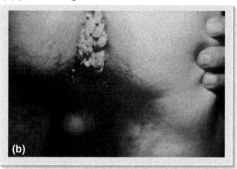

Source: CDC Public Health Image Library/Dr. M.F. Rein   Source: CDC Public Health Image Library/Dr. Wiesner

Table 21.2 Treatment of anogenital warts

Treatment	Description	Best suited to (wart morphology): Soft non-keratinised warts	Keratinised warts	Regimen	Advantages	Disadvantages
Cryotherapy	Physical ablative technique using liquid nitrogen (LN2) spray (−180°C) to freeze the skin resulting in cell cytolysis (breakdown)	(✓)*	✓	Freeze-thaw-freeze technique with a halo of freezing a few millimetres around the lesion, weekly for 4 – 6 weeks and review. If improving continue for a further 4 – 6 weeks	Can be used for visible urethra meatal warts; safe in pregnancy	Storage and handling safety issues with LN2 Patient discomfort Frequent appointments
Podophyllotoxin [Warticon®, Condylline®, Condylox® (USA)]	Antimitotic agent, purified extract of podophyllin, available in a cream (0.15%) or alcoholic solution (0.5%). Cream is easier to apply but less effective than the solution. Supervision by medical staff is recommended if treatment area > 4cm²	✓		Apply twice daily for 3 consecutive days followed by 4 days' rest, for 4 weekly cycles. Review	Patient can self-administer (home treat)	Use contraindicated in pregnancy and lactation; use for perianal lesions is 'off-licence'; not recommended for internal lesions; local side effects
Imiquimod (5%) cream (Aldara®)	Immune response modifier used for refractory warts or occasionally first-line if cryotherapy not available	✓	✓	Apply 3 times a week on non-consecutive days, and leave on skin for 6 – 10 hours (e.g. overnight) then wash off. 4 weekly reviews with up to a maximum of 16 weeks' treatment per episode of warts	Recurrence rates lower; Patient can self-administer (home treat)	Expensive (x 2 – 3 > podophyllotoxin) Not suitable for internal warts Contraindicated in pregnancy Skin reactions common and can be severe
Surgical excision	Removal of warts by excision under local anaesthetic. Haemostasis achieved with electrosurgery or silver nitrate		✓	Useful for pedunculated warts or small number of keratinised warts	Immediate cosmetic treatment, procedure can be repeated as necessary	Discomfort, scarring

* For a small number of low volume warts, irrespective of morphology, cryotherapy is commonly used first-line.
All treatments may involve discomfort and side-effects such as local skin reactions, ulceration and scarring. Podophyllotoxin and imiquimod cream may weaken latex condoms. Local anaesthetic cream can be used before ablative therapies to minimise discomfort

Sexual and Reproductive Health at a Glance, First Edition. Catriona Melville. © 2015 by John Wiley & Sons, Ltd. Published 2015 by John Wiley & Sons, Ltd.
Companion website: www.ataglanceseries.com/sexualhealth

Background

Anogenital human papilloma virus (HPV) is the most frequent sexually transmitted viral infection in the world. Anogenital warts (condylomata acuminata or genital warts) are responsible for substantial morbidity and healthcare costs.

Aetiology and epidemiology

- Anogenital warts are caused by the human papilloma virus (HPV) which causes a multifocal infection of the genital skin
- There are >100 different genotypes of this double stranded DNA virus; however, the 'low risk' (non-oncogenic) types 6 and 11 are responsible for about 90% of anogenital warts (Table 21.1)
- At least 13 types of HPV are 'high risk' or oncogenic. Oncogenic HPV types are responsible for almost all cervical squamous cell cancers, and for 90% of anal, at least 12% oropharyngeal and 40% of cancers of the external genitalia (penis, vulva, vagina)
- Most lesions are benign; however, some anogenital warts will be co-infected with oncogenic types of HPV
- Infection begins in the basal cells of the epithelium which progresses to abnormal cell proliferation at the skin surface (visible as a wart)
- Peak age incidence is 25–34 years in men and 20–24 years in women
- The median incubation period is 3 months; however, it can be shorter or considerably longer and this long latent period is important in advising individuals who have concerns about partner infidelity
- Studies have shown a prevalence of genital HPV of up to 50% of sexually active adults
- Smoking, hormonal factors (such as pregnancy) and immunosuppression are associated with an increased likelihood of HPV detection

Transmission

- Anogenital warts are mostly sexually transmitted via contact with genital lesions and/or genital secretions containing virus. Micro-abrasions in the recipient's skin allow viral access to the basal epithelial cells
- Transmission can occur with non-penetrative sex and orogenital contact. Occasionally digital to genital transmission can also occur. HPV can be transmitted perinatally. Digital warts in children can be transmitted to the genital region however sexual abuse must be considered in any child presenting with anogenital warts
- Perianal warts can develop without anal sex and are common in both genders, however occur more frequently in MSM. Warts in the anal canal may be associated with penetrative anal sex
- HPV is highly infectious and acquisition increases with the number of sexual partners. Transmission rates between partners is 60%
- Most HPV infections are subclinical; >90% of infected individuals will have no visible lesions (warts)
- Spontaneous regression occurs in 30% of individuals in 6 months and HPV DNA is no longer detectable in over 90% of individuals by 2 years post-infection

Symptoms and signs

Symptoms

- Most patients present with genital lump or growths
- Warts are usually not painful but can be associated with itch or irritation and can bleed (anal/cervical/urethral lesions)
- Urethral warts can cause distortion of the urinary stream

- Although physical symptoms of anogenital warts are usually minimal, individuals with the condition often find it extremely psychologically distressing

Signs

- Warts may be single or multiple, raised or flat (papular), keratinized or soft. They may be broad based or pedunculated, and skin coloured or pigmented (Figure 21.1)
- Keratinized warts tend to occur on the dry hair-bearing skin (e.g. labia majora, scrotum), whereas those on moist, warm areas tend to be soft and non-keratinized (e.g. vaginal introitus)
- Warts are usually <10 mm diameter but can coalesce into larger lesions
- There may be asymptomatic (occult) lesions on the cervix, vagina, urethral meatus, and anal canal
- Lesions can also be seen in extragenital sites e.g. oral cavity, larynx, conjunctivae, and nasal cavity

Diagnosis

- Differential diagnosis (Box 21.1)
- Diagnosis is based on clinical appearance (naked eye examination)
- Atypical/suspicious lesions should be biopsied under local anaesthetic
- Examination: use a good light to examine anogenital area. Perform a vaginal speculum in women
- Proctoscopy is not routinely performed in patients with external anogenital warts unless there are anorectal symptoms
- Document site(s), distribution, number and morphology of warts. A genital map can be helpful for recording this

Special situations

- Pregnancy: warts can appear or increase in size in pregnancy. The risk of the infant developing juvenile laryngeal papillomatosis is approximately 1 in 400 if warts are present at delivery. Treatment does not seem to diminish this risk and genital warts will often regress spontaneously in the puerperium. Cryotherapy can be offered. Imiquimod (not approved) and podophyllotoxin (possibly teratogenic) should not be used
- Immunosuppression, e.g. HIV infection and patients with diabetes have a poorer response to treatment and a higher relapse rate

Management (Table 21.2)

General

- The objective of treatment is removal of visible warts (cosmetic) rather than eradication of HPV
- As spontaneous resolution is likely to occur, no treatment is an option at any site
- Choice of treatment depends on the morphology, site and number of lesions, patient's preference and local protocols
- Treatment may take 1–6 months and there are significant failure and relapse rates with all treatments
- Smokers may respond less well to treatment than non-smokers
- 10–20% of individuals diagnosed with anogenital warts will have other STIs therefore STI testing should be offered

Treatment

- Commonly used treatment choices in the UK are listed in Table 21.2
- Intravaginal and intra-anal warts do not require treatment unless symptomatic

- Less commonly used therapies are trichloracetic acid (TCA), electrosurgery and laser treatment
- Women with anogenital warts should not change the frequency of cervical screening. Refer to colposcopy is there is clinical concern regarding cervical lesions

Follow-up and PN

- Tracing of previous sexual partners is not recommended
- Treatment of sexual partners makes no impact on the natural history of the index patient's infection however current partners can be offered STI screening and advice about the condition
- Data is conflicting; however, condom use may provide some protection against HPV acquisition and may have a therapeutic effect when both partners are infected, possibly by reducing continued re-exposure to the virus
- Patients with significant psychological distress may need referral for counselling

Vaccination

The UK, Australia and the USA have HPV vaccination programmes to help protect against cervical cancer. Gardasil®, a quadrivalent HPV vaccine (effective against HPV types 6, 11, 16, 18) has been in use in Australia since 2007 and was introduced in the UK in 2012. This appears to have had a substantial effect in reducing the clinical burden of genital warts.

Cervical Screening

- Cervical screening is a tool for detecting pre-malignant disease of the cervix. It has been shown to be an effective method of reducing the incidence and mortality of cervical cancer. In the UK, mortality rates from squamous cell cervical cancer have fallen by 7% a year since the introduction of the cervical screening call/recall programme in the 1980s
- UK call and recall schedule: Practice has differed across the UK until recently however the UK National Screening Committee has recommended that all screening should begin at aged 25 years (current practice in England and Northern Ireland)

First invitation (age) 25 years
Routine recall 3 yearly between 25 and 49 and then
  5 yearly until 65 years

- All cervical screening in the UK is done using liquid-based cytology technology which has several advantages over traditional cytology including less tests being reported as inadequate and a greater sensitivity than conventional cytology
- Dyskaryosis is a cytological diagnosis and can be reported as low grade or high grade (moderate, severe or query invasive squamous carcinoma)
- CIN is a histological diagnosis and is classified as stages 1–3 correlating with worsening dyskaryosis
- Technique (Figure 21.2): A speculum examination is used to visualize the cervix. The sample should be taken from the transformation zone (squamo-columnar junction). An endocervical brush is used to take the sample. The central bristles are inserted

into the endocervical canal and the brush is rotated five times in a clockwise direction. This is important to achieve a high cellular yield. Depending on the sampling kit used, the head of the brush should either be broken off into a vial of fixative (e.g. Surepath™), or rinsed in the vial using a vigorous swirling motion before pushing the brush against the bottom of the vial at least 10 ten times to force the bristles apart (Thinprep®)

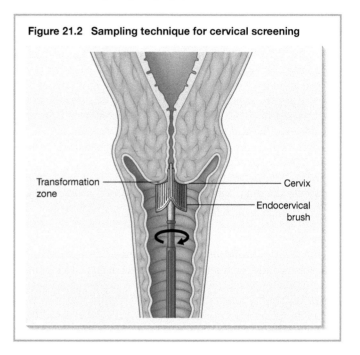

Figure 21.2 Sampling technique for cervical screening

HPV screening

Research has shown that women who have no cytological abnormalities and are HPV negative 6 months post-treatment for CIN can safely be returned to routine three yearly screening. In England pilot studies are underway to assess incorporating HPV testing into the cervical screening programme. In Scotland in 2012, HPV testing was introduced as a 'test of cure' for all women treated for CIN 1, 2 or 3. The HPV test is carried out on the sample taken for the cytology test.

Women with HIV

The prevalence of CIN and cervical HPV infection is high in HIV positive women. Cervical screening should therefore be carried out in all newly diagnosed women and continued on an annual basis. The age range should be the same as for HIV negative women. An initial colposcopy is also recommended if resources permit.

Pregnancy

Routine screening should be deferred in pregnancy. If the previous test was abnormal and pregnancy occurs in the interim, then the test should not be delayed, but should be taken in mid-trimester unless there is a clinical contraindication.

22 Genital infestations

Figure 22.1 Crab louse

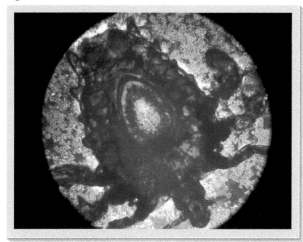

Microscopy x100 magnification
Source: Mark Mason, Senior Specialist Biomedical Scientist, Sandyford, NHS Greater Glasgow & Clyde, Glasgow, UK. Reproduced with permission of Sandyford.

Pediculosis pubis (Figure 22.1)

Background

Pediculosis pubis – also known as pubic lice – is an infestation caused by the crab louse *Phthirus pubis*. This is a different species from the one that causes head lice. The adult louse adheres to course hairs such as pubic hair, body hair (including beards), and less commonly eyebrows and eyelashes. *Phthirus pubis* is a blood-sucking insect. It is round, approximately 1–2 mm long and dark grey/brown in colour.

• *Life cycle*: the incubation period is 5 days to 5 weeks. The adult female lays eggs (nits) at the base of the hairs which usually hatch within 7 days. The eggs are strongly adherent to the hairs
• *Transmission*: is by close body contact. The louse requires a human host to survive and is unlikely to endure for much longer than 24 hours off the host

Signs and symptoms

• Pruritis, especially of the genital area is the commonest symptom. The itch is caused by hypersensitivity to the faeces and saliva of the lice
• Infection may be asymptomatic or the individual may notice nits or lice on their body
• Small blue macules – maculae caeruleae – caused by bleeding into the skin at feeding sites may be seen

Diagnosis

• The condition is diagnosed by finding adult lice and or nits on body hair. Naked eye examination usually suffices; however, low-power light microscopy can be used to view suspected lice or eggs

Management

• *General*: an STI screen should be offered. Clothes and bed linen should be washed at 50°C. Close body contact should be avoided until the index patient and partner(s) have been treated

• *Recommended treatments*: aqueous preparations and dermal cream are preferred over alcoholic preparations as the latter can irritate excoriated skin. A second application is advisable after 7 days
  – Malathion 0.5% aqueous solution applied over the whole body and washed off after at least 2 hours (preferably 12 hours) OR
  – Permethrin 5% cream rinse applied over the whole body and washed off after 12 hours. Treatment of choice in pregnancy or breastfeeding
• *Treatment of eyelashes*: Permethrin 1% lotion can be applied to closed eyes for 10 minutes. Alternatively, to avoid any eye irritation, soft paraffin eye ointment can be applied to lashes and eyelash roots BD for 8–10 days to suffocate the adult lice and nymphs (immature lice)
• *Partner notification*: current partners and those within the preceding 3 months should be examined and treated
• *Follow-up*: re-examine 1 week after final treatment and if live lice present try an alternative therapy. Dead nits may still be adherent to hairs. These can be removed with a nit comb. Individuals should be reassured that pruritis may persist for a week or more after successful treatment. Antihistamines can be helpful in managing this

Genital scabies (Figure 22.2)

Background

This infestation is caused by a parasitic mite, *Sarcoptes scabiei*. The female mites burrow into the skin and lay one to three eggs daily during their lifespan (4–6 weeks). The larvae hatch in 3–4 days, crawling out onto the skin and making new burrows. The mites feed on lymph and lysed skin tissue. Mites can only survive for a maximum of 72 hours when separated from the host

Figure 22.2 Scabies mite

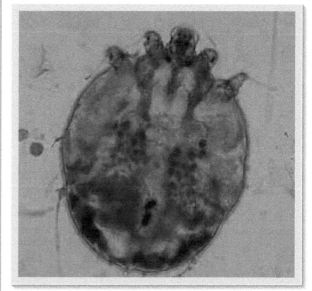

Microscopy x100 magnification
Source: Mark Mason, Senior Specialist Biomedical Scientist, Sandyford, NHS Greater Glasgow & Clyde, Glasgow, UK. Reproduced with permission of Sandyford.

Sexual and Reproductive Health at a Glance, First Edition. Catriona Melville. © 2015 by John Wiley & Sons, Ltd. Published 2015 by John Wiley & Sons, Ltd.
Companion website: www.ataglanceseries.com/sexualhealth

- Transmission: is by skin-to-skin contact (mites are transferred after about 10–20 minutes of close contact) but not necessarily sexually transmitted as it can affect any part of the body, e.g. can be transmitted from hand holding

Signs and symptoms

- Generalized pruritis, especially at night is caused by the absorption of mite excrement into skin capillaries causing a hypersensitivity reaction. Secondary infection can occur from excoriation
- Genital papules or nodules may be seen or silvery lines in the skin where mites have burrowed
- Classical sites are the interdigital folds, wrists, extensor surfaces of elbows, genitals and around the nipples in women

Diagnosis

- A clinical diagnosis is usually made from the typical signs and symptoms. Scrapings can be taken from burrows and examined under light microscopy to reveal mites. The appearance can be confused with eczema

Management

- *General*: An STI screen should be offered if sexual acquisition is likely. Clothes and bed linen should be washed at ≥50°C. Close body contact should be avoided until the index patient and partner(s)/close household members have been treated
- *Treatment*: Permethrin 5% dermal cream (safe in breastfeeding or pregnancy) or Malathion 0.5% aqueous solution applied to the whole body from the neck down and washed off after 12 hours (permethrin) or 24 hours (Malathion). Repeat treatment after 7 days. Itch may persist for several weeks after successful treatment. Antihistamines can be helpful in managing symptoms
- *Partner notification*: trace and treat current household and sexual contacts and those within the preceding 2 months
- *Follow-up*: re-treat if new burrows appear
- Norwegian scabies is a variant which occurs in the immunocompromised (e.g. HIV infection) or the elderly. Hyperkeratotic crusting lesions occur which are teeming with thousands of mites. It is highly contagious. This condition is treated with Ivermectin 200 µg/kg (on a named patient basis)

23 Anogenital dermatoses

Figure 23.1 Lichen sclerosus

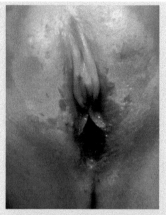

Treatment regimen
Ultra-potent topical steroid applied
- Once a day for 1 month
  then
- Alternate days for 1 month
  then
- Twice weekly for 1 month
  then review

Source: CDC Public Health Image Library/Joe Miller

Figure 23.2 Lichen planus

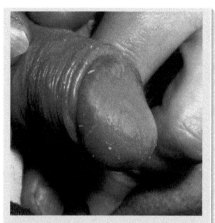

Treatment regimen
Ultra-potent topical steroid applied
- Once a day for 1 month
  then
- Alternate days for 1 month
  then
- Twice weekly for 1 month
  then review

Source: CDC Public Health Image Library/Susan Lindsley; Donated by Brian Hill, New Zealand

Figure 23.3 Psoriasis of the buttocks and natal cleft

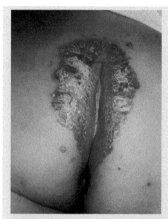

Management
- Avoid irritants and use emollient soap substitute
- Topical corticosteroid (strength depending on disease severity) ± antifungal or antibiotic agent as indicated
- Coal-tar preparations
- Vitamin D analogues, e.g. Talcalcitol

Source: CDC Public Health Image Library/Dr. Gavin Hart

Table 23.1 Causes of balanitis

Infections (STI and non-STI)	*Candida albicans*, TV, streptococci, anaerobes, *Gardnerella vaginalis, Staphylococcus aureus,* syphilis, HSV, HPV
Dermatoses	LS, LP, psoriasis, contact allergy, plasma cell (Zoon's) balanitis, circinate balanitis, Stevens-Johnson Syndrome, fixed drug eruption
Miscellaneous	Trauma, poor hygiene, pre-malignant conditions, irritants e.g. soaps

Figure 23.4 VIN

Management of VIN
- Local excision of affected tissue
- Imiquimod cream 5% (unlicensed indication)
- Vulvectomy

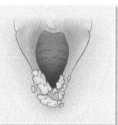

Figure 23.5 PIN

- PIN is also known as Bowen disease of the penis or erythroplasia of Queyrat
- Uncircumcised men > 50 years are most at risk
- May resemble balanitis or psoriasis, with erythema, itching, crusting or ulcers
- 10 – 30% cases progress to invasive squamous cell carcinoma without treatment
- Investigations: suspicious lesions should be biopsied
- Treatment: local excision; Imiquimod 5%, laser therapy, 5-fluorouracil cream

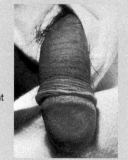

Source: CDC Public Health Image Library/Susan Lindsley

Box 23.1 Topical calcineurine inhibitors

- Tacrolimus and pimecrolimus are immunomodulating agents which have an anti-inflammatory effect
- Licensed for use in atopic eczema and also used for LS, LP and psoriasis (unlicensed)
- They do not cause skin atrophy (c.f. topical steroids), however local skin irritation is common
- No long-term safety data is available
- Use is contraindicated in pregnancy

Box 23.2 Genital skin care advice

Important for the management of all dermatoses.
- Avoid contact with soap, shampoo, shower gel and bubble bath
- Use simple emollients as a soap substitute and general moisturiser e.g. aqueous cream BP, diprobase, soft paraffin. Emollients can also be added to bath water
- Avoid tight-fitting garments which may irritate the area. Loose-fitting cotton underwear may help
- Wearing cotton gloves at night and using an anti-histamine can help manage night-time scratching
- Textile dyes in coloured toilet paper or underwear can be irritant

Box 23.3 Balanitis

Balanitis is inflammation of the glans penis which in uncircumcised males usually occurs together with inflammation of the prepuce (posthitis) as balanoposthitis.

- Symptoms: rash, itch, odour, dysuria
- Signs: erythema, purpura, fissuring, oedema, odour phimosis
- Investigations: subpreputial swab for candida and other bacteria (if present test for diabetes with fasting blood sugar); PCR for HSV/syphilis if ulceration; STI screen if indicated; biopsy if suspicious lesions
- Management: treat underlying cause if identified. Genital hygiene advice (Box 23.2), avoid over-washing (Table 23.1)

Lichen sclerosus (LS)

- Aetiology: inflammatory condition of unknown cause. Linked to autoimmune disorders. Occurs 10 times more commonly in women than men and although it can present at any age (including children), it is predominantly seen in women >50 years. In men LS is known as balanitis xerotica obliterans (BXO)
- Complications: risk of development of squamous cell carcinoma is unknown but thought to be <5%
- Symptoms: itch, irritation, soreness and dyspareunia (due to introital narrowing). Rarely asymptomatic
- Signs: females; skin pallor or atrophy ('cigarette paper' appearance) either in patches or in a 'figure of eight' distribution (involving perianal area). Hyperkeratosis, fissuring, excoriation and purpura (ecchymosis). Loss of architecture with labial adhesions and midline fusion may be seen; males; affects the glans penis. Scarring can cause obliteration of the urethral meatus
- Diagnosis: is clinical unless uncertainty or malignancy suspected in which case a biopsy is required
- Investigations: screen for other autoimmune conditions if indicated, e.g. thyroid disease. Take a skin swab if secondary infection is suspected
- Management: there is no cure for LS and it usually persists for years. Treatment can substantially improve symptoms. Mainstay is ultra-potent topical steroids e.g. clobetasol proprionate. A 30-g tube should last 3 months. Ointment bases are preferable to creams
- Follow-up: review in 2–3 months. Maintenance treatment may be required. Stable disease should be reviewed annually however individuals should be advised to seek advice if they notice any suspicious changes (e.g. raised lesions) (see Figure 23.1)

Lichen planus (LP)

- Aetiology: uncommon inflammatory condition of unknown cause. LP is linked to autoimmune disorders. It can affect the skin, genital and oral mucous membranes. It occurs equally in men and women and can present at any age. In the majority of cases (85%), it resolves within 18 months
- Symptoms: itch, irritation, soreness, vaginal discharge, or dyspareunia or can be asymptomatic
- Signs: females; there are different subtypes of LP. Erosive LP is the commonest type affecting the vulva. It can also affect the vagina (unlike LS). The mucosal surfaces are eroded, The erosion edges are purple with a pale network of fine white lines – Wickham's striae. As the erosions heal, synaechiae and scarring can develop. Lesions of classical LP can be found on the keratinized anogenital skin as can hypertrophic lesions. In males; lesions of the glans penis may occur
- Complications: scarring, including vaginal synechiae formation. Risk of development of squamous cell carcinoma may be as high as 3%
- Diagnosis: clinical or biopsy and histology if uncertain
- Investigations: as per LS
- Management: Is similar to LS, with ultra-potent topical steroids, e.g. clobetasol proprionate. Maintenance treatment may be necessary and can be with weaker steroids or with less frequent use of ultra-potent steroids. Intravaginal corticosteroid treatments may be indicated
- Follow-up: as per LS (see Figure 23.2)

Dermatitis

Can be atopic, allergic contact, irritant contact or seborrhoeic. Dermatitis can be secondary to iron deficiency anaemia or candidal infection.

- Symptoms: itch, soreness
- Signs: lichenification, excoriation, fissuring, erythema
- Diagnosis: clinical, general examination to look for skin disease elsewhere
- Investigations: patch testing and biopsy if indicated, swab for infection (especially candida), serum ferritin
- Management: avoid precipitating factors. Topical steroids (choice determined by disease severity). Combination preparations with antifungal +/or antibiotic for superinfection. Emollients and soap substitutes. Topical calcineurine inhibitors (Box 23.1)
- Complications: secondary infection

Lichen simplex

LS is a localized dermatitis caused by repeated rubbing and scratching inducing a chronic itch–scratch cycle. The stimulus to scratch may be an existing skin condition, e.g. atopic dermatitis; a systemic condition associated with pruritis, e.g. primary biliary cirrhosis; or environmental factors, e.g heat, sweat. It is also associated with psychiatric disorders such as anxiety, depression and obsessive-compulsive disorder.

- Symptoms: itch, soreness
- Signs: can affect the anal or genital skin in both males (e.g. scrotum) and females (e.g. labia majora). Lichenification, erosions and fissuring, excoriation
- Diagnosis: clinical
- Complications: secondary infections
- Investigations: swab for infection, consider patch testing, serum ferritin, and biopsy if indicated
- Management: avoid precipitating factors, use emollients, topical corticosteroid, antihistamine at night, and address any mental health issues

Psoriasis

- Aetiology: a common, chronic skin condition affecting about 2% of the population. It affects adult men and women in equal proportions and has a genetic predisposition. Genital psoriasis may present as part of plaque or flexural psoriasis or be the only area affected (rare); 5% of sufferers will develop psoriatic arthritis
- Symptoms: itch, soreness
- Signs: well demarcated erythematous scaly plaques, fissuring, often symmetrical. Natal cleft involvement common
- Complications: Koebner effect (skin lesions appearing at sites of trauma)
- Diagnosis: typical clinical appearance. Examine for lesions elsewhere (see Figure 23.3)

Premalignant conditions

The commonest aetiology of vulval, penile and anal intraepithelial neoplasia (VIN, PIN, AIN) is HPV (especially type 16) but they are also associated with LS, smoking and immunosuppression. Clinical appearance can be variable ranging from atypical warty lesions to raised erythematous or pigmented lesions. Multifocal lesions are common. They can cause itch, pain and burning or be asymptomatic. VIN is associated with CIN therefore up to date cytology should be confirmed ± colposcopy. Diagnosis is histological. Progression to squamous cell carcinoma can occur in 9–18.5% of VIN. Management in a multidisciplinary vulval clinic is recommended (see Figures 23.4 and 23.5).

24 # Viral hepatitis A, B and C

Table 24.1 Summary of hepatitis A, B and C

Virus	Hepatitis A RNA virus (Picorna)	Hepatitis B DNA virus (Hepadna)	Hepatitis C RNA virus (Flaviviridae)
Transmission routes	Faecal–oral (usual), sexual (infrequent)	Parenteral, vertical, sexual	Parenteral, vertical, sexual
Incubation period	15 – 45 days	40 – 160 days	4 – 20 weeks
Infectious period	From 2 weeks before until 1 week after the onset of jaundice	From 2 weeks before jaundice until sAg negative (may take up to 6 months)	From 2 weeks before jaundice (if there was no acute infection trace back to the likely time of infection, e.g. first needle sharing)
Carrier state/ chronic infection	None	5 – 10% adults	50 – 85%
Vaccine	Yes	Yes*	No
Vaccination schedule	• 0 then 6 – 12 months • 95% protection for 10 years (possibly lifelong) Vaccination should be offered to certain groups of individuals (Box 24.1)	• Ultra-rapid regimen: 0, 7, 12 days, 12 months • Rapid regimen: 0, 1, 2, 12 months • Standard regimen: 0, 1, 6 months • Full primary course confers lifelong immunity in healthy individuals	N/A
Pregnancy and breastfeeding	• No teratogenic effects • Increased rate of miscarriage and premature labour in acute infection • Vertical transmission reported but extremely rare • Breastfeeding can continue	• Risk of vertical transmission: 90% if mother is HBeAg-positive; 10% if HBeAg negative • > 90% of infected infants become chronic carriers • Vaccination at birth reduces vertical transmission by 90% • Breastfeeding has no additional transmission risk so can continue	• Risk of vertical transmission is low (approx 5%) but higher if HIV +ve • Increased rate of miscarriage and premature labour in acute infection • Breastfeeding can continue unless cracked or bleeding nipples
Diagnosis (serology)	HAV IgM (remains positive for 6 months or more)	See Table 24.2	• Hep C Ab (may take 3 months to become positive) • HCV-RNA (antigen test) will be positive after 2 weeks**
Partner notification	Sexual contacts (MSM and other at-risk contacts) during infectious period should be reviewed and offered hepatitis A vaccination up to 14 days post-exposure (if exposure was in the infectious period). Human normal immunoglobulin (HNIG) 250 – 500 mg can be considered for contacts at higher risk of complications, e.g. chronic liver disease. Its efficacy is highest in the first few days after contact and benefits unlikely after 14 days post-exposure. Household contacts are managed by public health authorities	• Sexual and needle sharing contacts from during infectious period should be reviewed and offered vaccination Non-immune contacts can be offered specific hepatitis B immunoglobulin 500 i.u. i.m. (HBIG). This is most effective within 48 hours of a single exposure and is of no use > 7 days post-exposure. An accelerated course of vaccine should also be offered to those given HBIG (and all sexual and household contacts). • HBV PEP may be required following sexual or occupational exposure. (e.g. needlestick injury, mucous membrane splash)	• Sexual and needle sharing contacts from during infectious period should be reviewed and tested • Discuss sexual transmission. Consistent use of condoms should avoid onwards transmission • There is no PEP or vaccine available for HCV
Comments		* Vaccination should be offered to non-immune individuals in at-risk groups (Box 24.2). Rapid schedules have better compliance than standard vaccination regimens. If a course of immunization is interrupted it can be resumed rather than restarted. Post-vaccination titres are no longer routinely recommended. • HBV is the most infectious BBV	** Ab test indicates exposure to the virus; chronic infection confirmed if HCV-RNA +ve 6 months after first positive test

Box 24.1 Vaccination for hepatitis A

Injecting drug users (PWD) Occupational risk
MSM Chronic liver diseases (including HCV)
Travellers to endemic countries Haemophiliacs

Box 24.2 Hepatitis B testing (in sexual health) should be offered to:

• Individuals from countries with a high prevalence of HBV e.g. Asia, Africa, Eastern Europe, Caribbean
• Men who have sex with men (and are not already immunised)
• Individuals who have been sexually assaulted
• Male and female sex workers
• Sexual partners of positive or at risk individuals
• Injecting drug users
• Individuals diagnosed with HIV or HCV
• Needle-stick victims, individuals with unsterile tattoos or piercings

Box 24.3 Hepatitis C testing

• People who have ever injected drugs
• People who received blood products or organ transplant before Sep 1991
• Following a needle-stick injury if the donor HCV status is positive or unknown
• Those with known HIV or HBV infection
• Children born to HCV positive women (deferred until aged 12 months)
• Sexual partners of those at risk of or living with Hepatitis C
• People who may have had unsterile body piercing, tattooing or acupuncture
• People who may have had unsterile medical or dental procedures abroad

Table 24.2 HBV serology

Serological marker (notes)	Acute infection	Chronic infection	Previous resolved infection (naturally immune)	Successful vaccination
HBcAb (anti-core antibody) Marker of acquired infection; positive in resolved infection (persists for life); negative in vaccinated patients	Negative (unless late or symptomatic acute infection)	Positive	Positive	Negative
HBsAg (surface antigen) Positive in acute and chronic infection Disappears in resolved infection	Positive	Positive	Negative	Negative
HBeAg (envelope antigen) Marker of high viral activity (= infectivity)	Positive	Positive (high infectivity) or Negative	Negative	Negative
Anti-HBs (anti-surface antibody) Marker of successful vaccination Titres determine level of protection	Negative	Negative	Positive	Positive

Sexual and Reproductive Health at a Glance, First Edition. Catriona Melville. © 2015 by John Wiley & Sons, Ltd. Published 2015 by John Wiley & Sons, Ltd.
Companion website: www.ataglanceseries.com/sexualhealth

Background

Viral hepatitis is a group of infectious diseases affecting hundreds of millions of people globally. Five distinct viruses have been identified: A, B C, D and E. Hepatitis A, B and C in the context of SRH will be reviewed in this chapter.

Acute viral hepatitis infection is often asymptomatic and therefore widely under-diagnosed. In the UK it causes a significant public health burden. Acute viral hepatitis is a notifiable disease in England and Wales, and hepatitis A, B and C are notifiable organisms in Scotland.

Hepatitis A (Table 24.1, Box 24.1)

Hepatitis A virus (HAV) is common in developing countries with poor sanitation. It is excreted in the stools and usually spread though ingestion of contaminated food or water or direct contact with an infectious person. In endemic regions, it largely affects children. It is less common in developed countries, where it can cause disease in any age group. It can be transmitted sexually by oro-anal or digital-rectal contact. Outbreaks have been reported in MSM in the UK however seroprevalence studies have shown similar rates of HAV antibodies in heterosexual and homosexual men.

Symptoms and signs

- Up to 50% of adults and most children will have no symptoms, or mild non-specific symptoms with little or no jaundice
- Symptoms include a prodromal illness with flu-like symptoms, pyrexia and right upper abdominal pain lasting 3–10 days followed by an icteric illness with jaundice, nausea and fatigue (1–3 weeks)
- Signs: jaundice, pale stools and dark urine, hepatomegaly and dehydration

Complications

- 15% of cases will require hospitalization and approximately 0.4% of cases will be complicated by acute liver failure (ALF). HAV associated mortality is extremely low (<0.1%)

Management

- General: information and advice about condition. Advise no food handling or UPSI until non-infectious
- Investigations: LFTs and coagulation factors, serology for other hepatitis viruses, HIV and syphilis. Screen for other STIs if sexually acquired hepatitis
- Most cases are managed supportively as outpatients, however if Prothrombin time (PT) prolonged by >5 seconds, or severe dehydration or signs of hepatic decompensation occur then admit to hospital Follow-up at 2 weekly intervals until LFTs are normal

Hepatitis B (Tables 24.1, 24.2, Box 24.2)

Hepatitis B virus (HBV) is endemic globally with 240 million people suffering from chronic infection worldwide. In the UK the seroprevalence is 0.01–0.04% in blood donors, but >1% in people who inject drugs (PWIDs) and MSM. It can be transmitted parenterally (e.g. blood products, sharing infected needles or 'works', needle-stick injuries, tattoos), vertically or sexually. Sexual transmission occurs in unvaccinated MSM and correlates with multiple partners, unprotected anal sex and oro-anal sex ('rimming'). Transmission also occurs after heterosexual contact. Sex workers are at higher risk of acquiring the infection. Chronic infection is defined as >6 months HBsAg positive.

Symptoms and signs

- Acute phase: nearly all infants and children and 10–50% of adults (especially if HIV co-infection) are asymptomatic

- Prodromal and icteric symptoms are similar to HAV but may be more severe. With the exception of fatigue and loss of appetite, chronic carriers are usually symptomless
- Signs in acute HBV are similar to HAV. In chronic infection after many years, signs of chronic liver disease may be apparent, e.g. finger clubbing, jaundice, ascites

Complications

- <1% of acute cases develop fulminant hepatitis
- Chronic infection is more common in the immune-compromised including HIV; 10–50% of chronic carriers will develop liver cirrhosis and ≥10% of cirrhotic patients will progress to liver cancer. Concurrent infection with HCV can lead to more progressive liver disease

Management

- General: avoid UPSI until they are non-infectious or their partners have been successfully vaccinated
- Investigations and management of acute infection: as for HAV. Liver biopsy and further imaging may be indicated. Patients with chronic infection should be managed by a hepatologist
- Follow-up as per acute HAV but repeat serology after 6 months to exclude chronic infection
- Antiviral therapies and interferon are licensed for use in chronic infection

Screening (Box 24.2, Table 24.2)

Anti-HBc and/or HBsAg are often used for screening. If both are negative then there is no evidence of past or current infection and vaccination should be offered if applicable. If Anti-HBc is positive but HBsAg is negative then the patient is naturally immune and no further action is required. If HBsAg is also positive, the patient has current infection (either acute or chronic).

Hepatitis C (Table 24.1, Box 24.3)

Hepatitis C virus (HCV) is endemic worldwide, and is the commonest BBV in the UK. The UK adult prevalence is approximately 0.5% but increases to >40% in PWID's (and >60% in PWID's in Scotland). In the UK the two major routes of transmission of HCV have been sharing of drug injecting equipment by PWIDs and transfusion of infected blood or blood products (pre-1990s). Sexual transmission occurs at a low rate but is increased if the index patient is HIV co-infected.

Symptoms and signs

The majority of patients undergo asymptomatic acute infection (>70–80%). Symptoms and signs of acute icteric hepatitis are similar to HAV. Chronic carriers are usually asymptomatic or may have non-specific ill health. Signs of chronic infection are similar to HBV.

Complications

- <1% of acute cases develop fulminant hepatitis
- Up to one-third of chronic carriers will progress to severe liver disease after 14–30 years. Cirrhosis develops in 20–30% after 20 years and there is an increased risk of liver cancer

Management

- Advise patient not to donate blood/semen/organs. Toothbrushes, razors and needles should not be shared and alcohol should be avoided
- Further investigations as per HAV
- High-dose α-interferon or pegylated interferon reduces the rate of chronicity to ≤10%. Liver biopsy and further imaging may be indicated. All patients with active infection should be referred to a specialist centre

25 HIV

Figure 25.1 HIV virus

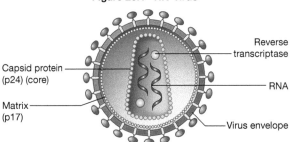

Capsid protein (p24) (core)

Matrix (p17)

Reverse transcriptase

RNA

Virus envelope

Figure 25.2 Natural history of untreated HIV infection

Acute HIV infection
- Glandular fever-type illness
- Seroconversion occurs

Clinical latency
- 5 – 10 years (variable)
- Gradual decline in CD4 count and increase in HIV RNA without treatment

Symptomatic HIV infection
- The immune system becomes severely damaged by HIV and symptoms develop without treatment, e.g. lymphadenopathy, seborrhoeic dermatitis, fever

AIDs
- Opportunistic infections
- CD4 count < 200 cells/µl
- Without treatment survival is typically 3 years

Table 25.1 Risk of HIV transmission following exposure

Type of exposure	Risk of HIV transmission (median %) following a single exposure from a known HIV-positive source
Sexual intercourse:	
• Receptive anal intercourse	1.11%
• Insertive anal intercourse	0.06%
• Receptive vaginal intercourse	0.1%
• Insertive vaginal intercourse	0.08%
• Receptive oral sex (giving fellatio)	0.02%
• Insertive oral sex (receiving fellatio or cunnilingus)	Unknown but close to zero
Sharing injecting drug equipment	0.7%
Blood transfusion (single unit)	90 – 100%
Occupational: needle-stick injury	0.3%

The probability of HIV transmission is also influenced by other factors e.g. high plasma viral load, breaches in mucosal barrier, whether ejaculation occurs, presence of concurrent STIs (which can enhance HIV shedding in the genital tract), aggravated sexual intercourse, e.g. sexual assault.

Box 25.1 Examples of AIDs-defining conditions

Pneumocystis jiroveci pneumonia (PCP)

Tuberculosis

Kaposi's sarcoma

Non-Hodgkins lymphoma

Oesophageal candida

Cerebral toxoplasmosis

Cytomegalovirus (CMV) retinitis

Mycobacterium avium Intracellulare

For full list see Center for Disease Control and Prevention (CDC), United States www.cdc.gov/hiv/

Figure 25.3 Oral conditions associated with symptomatic HIV infection: (a) oral candidiasis, (b) Intraoral Kaposi's sarcoma, (c) oral hairy leukoplakia

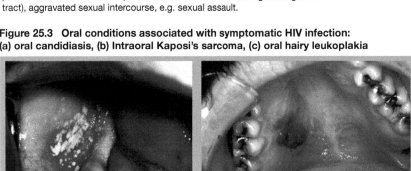
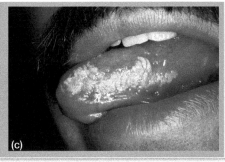

(a) (b) (c)

Source: CDC Public Health Image Library/Sol Silverman, Jr., D.D.S.

Source: CDC Public Health Image Library/J.S. Greenspan, B.D.S., University of California, San Francisco; Sol Silverman, Jr., D.D.S.

Sexual and Reproductive Health at a Glance, First Edition. Catriona Melville. © 2015 by John Wiley & Sons, Ltd. Published 2015 by John Wiley & Sons, Ltd.
Companion website: www.ataglanceseries.com/sexualhealth

Background

Human immunodeficiency virus (HIV) was first detected in 1983 in a patient with acquired immunodeficiency syndrome (AIDs). The infection is a major global public health issue with 35.3 million people living with HIV worldwide in 2012. Although incurable, HIV is treatable and prompt diagnosis and treatment improves clinical outcomes. In the UK an estimated 98,400 people were living with HIV in 2012. The majority of infected individuals in the UK are male (70%)

- *Aetiology*: HIV belongs to a group of retroviruses called lentiviruses. It is spherical and consists of an envelope, matrix and core (Figure 25.1). There are two types of HIV, the predominant type, HIV-1 and the less common HIV-2. HIV-1 is further subdivided into subtypes
- *Pathogenesis*: The virus causes depletion of CD4 lymphocytes (T helper cells). Over time there is progressive damage to the immune system leading to severe immune deficiency, opportunistic infections (OIs), cancers, and ultimately death if untreated (Figure 25.2). The most advanced stage of HIV infection is AIDs which can take from 2–15 years to develop. Not everyone with HIV will progress to AIDS. Early diagnosis and appropriate treatment can result in a near normal life expectancy
- *Transmission*: The virus is found in blood and body fluids (semen, vaginal fluid and breast milk). The routes of transmission are:
  - Sexual: unprotected anal, vaginal or oral (uncommon) sex
  - Sharing injecting equipment in PWIDs or in countries where sterile equipment is not available
  - Transfusion of infected blood and blood products. Blood has been screened for HIV in the UK since 1984
  - Vertical: from mother to child (antepartum, intrapartum or postpartum)
  - Occupational exposure: e.g. needle-stick injuries

The majority of infections are acquired sexually, with MSM and individuals from sub-Saharan Africa being disproportionately affected in the UK. The risks of transmission following a single exposure with HIV infection are listed in Table 25.1. The actual risk depends upon the type of exposure and the likelihood of the source being HIV positive. See PEP and PEPSE for further information (see Chapter 26).

Primary HIV infection (PHI)

Also known as HIV seroconversion illness, this usually occurs 2–6 weeks after infection. Symptoms develop in >60% of individuals however these are often non-specific and transient, e.g. pyrexia, sore throat, myalgia, fatigue and lymphadenopathy. Symptoms last 5–10 days although fatigue may persist. A maculopapular skin rash may develop, particularly on the trunk, and mucosal ulceration of the mouth or anogenital areas may occur. It can be confused with glandular fever (Epstein–Barr virus), other viral infections and primary syphilis.

- During the PHI virus replicates rapidly, and this is the stage of highest infectivity of HIV infection
- The CD4 count can fall rapidly (temporarily) and therefore conditions associated with immune deficiency may occur e.g. oral candidiasis, shingles
- Diagnosis at this early stage allows early identification of any partners at risk, thus minimising onwards transmission. It also enables early monitoring of viral load and administering antiretroviral therapy where clinically appropriate. If the diagnosis is missed at this stage then it may be several years before the individual presents to health services

Asymptomatic HIV infection

Following the symptoms of PHI the individual may remain well for many years. The CD4 count declines annually at a rate of approximately 40–80 cells/mm^3 (variable).

Symptomatic HIV infection

As the disease progresses untreated, opportunistic infections (OIs) develop (Figure 25.3). Fungi, bacteria and viruses can all cause OIs. This stage of HIV infection is often associated with constitutional symptoms, e.g. night sweats, malaise, diarrhoea and weight loss. Oral hairy leukoplakia, shingles or recurrent episodes of seborrhoeic dermatitis may occur.

Symptomatic (AIDs-defining) HIV infection

Certain infections, conditions and malignancies are classified as AIDs defining conditions (Box 25.1).

Diagnosis and investigations

Diagnosis/screening tests

- The p24 Ag is usually detected in 2–6 weeks. It becomes undetectable as antibodies develop. Antibodies to HIV can take 4–6 weeks to develop, but occasionally up to 12 weeks
- The first line serological assay is one which tests for p24 antigen and HIV antibody simultaneously (a so-called fourth generation test). This type of test performed in a laboratory will detect the majority of individuals who have been infected with HIV at 4 weeks after specific exposure
- The window period for HIV testing has traditionally been 12 weeks however in light of these latest technologies, BASHH and EAGA (the Expert Advisory Group on AIDs) recommend that a negative result on a fourth generation test performed at 4 weeks post-exposure is highly likely to exclude HIV infection. A further test at 8 weeks is recommended only following an event assessed as carrying a high risk of infection
- Patients who attend within 4 weeks of potential exposure should be offered testing at presentation and a repeat test at 4 weeks following the specific risk
- A positive HIV test should undergo confirmatory assays, and testing on a second sample arranged
- Rapid point of care testing (POCT); traditional testing relies on processing of a venous blood sample. POCT utilize a finger-prick or mouth swab sample and can offer a result within minutes. They are useful where venepuncture is not possible, e.g. outreach settings and/poor venous access or where an (almost) immediate result is advantageous. POCT have lower positive predictive value than traditional serological tests therefore all positive results must be confirmed on serological samples. Home testing kits can be sold 'over the counter' in the UK following a legislative change in April 2014

Investigations for evaluating and monitoring disease

- Viral load tests are quantitative HIV RNA assays. They are not usually used for diagnosis of HIV unless PHI is suspected and the HIV-Ab/p24Ag test is negative. Viral load reflects the rate of viral replication and can range from undetectable (<50 copies/mL) to over a million copies/ml. They are measured using a log 10 scale, e.g. 106 copies/ml. When the viral load is suppressed (i.e. by ART), the CD4 count can recover
- CD4 count is a measure of the degree of immunosuppression. In HIV-negative individuals it is usually 600–1200 per mm^3. The CD4 count helps guide when to start antiretroviral therapy (ART) and when to recommend prophylaxis against OIs

Box 25.2 HIV testing should be offered to the following individuals:

- All individuals diagnosed with an STI
- Men and women who have had UPSI (anal or vaginal)
- Sexual contacts of those diagnosed with HIV infection
- MSM and their female sexual contacts
- Individuals who have ever injected drugs
- Individuals diagnosed with a BBV
- Children of women who have HIV
- Individuals from a country with high HIV prevalence (> 1%) and their sexual contacts
- Individuals who have had sexual contact in a country with high HIV prevalence (> 1%)
- Anyone who has symptoms or conditions that could be associated with HIV infection (Table 25.1)

Box 25.3 HIV pre-test discussion

The pre-test discussion should encompass the following issues:

- The benefits of testing: early diagnosis associated with better prognosis; treatment, monitoring and support available
- Details of how the result will be given

Other issues which may be discussed are:

- The individual's understanding of HIV/AIDs
- The window period and need for repeat testing
- Confidentiality and legal issues (e.g. insurance)
- The individual's support network and ability to cope

Table 25.2 Conditions in adults associated with HIV infection ('HIV indicator conditions')

- Any lymphadenopathy of unknown cause
- Any unexplained blood dyscrasia including: thrombocytopenia, neutropenia, lymphopenia
- Pyrexia of unknown origin
- Mononucleosis-like illness, where EBV testing is negative
- Chronic diarrhoea of unknown cause
- Weight loss of unknown cause
- Cervical cancer and CIN Grade 2 or above

- Oral candidiasis
- Lymphoma
- Recurrent herpes zoster (or affecting multiple dermatomes)
- Recurrent bacterial infections e.g. pneumonia
- Chronic, recurrent salmonella, shigella or campylobacter infections
- Severe recalcitrant psoriasis
- Severe seborrhoeic dermatitis
- TB

For further information refer to: UK National Guidelines for HIV Testing 2008, British HIV Association, British Association of Sexual Health and HIV, British Infection Society, London. (http://www.bhiva.org/documents/Guidelines/Testing/GlinesHIVTest08.pdf)

Table 25.3 Main classes of antiretroviral drugs (ART)

Nucleoside/nucleotide reverse transcriptase inhibitors (NRTIs, NtRTIs)
Non-nucleoside reverse transcriptase inhibitors (NNRTIs)
Protease inhibitors (PIs)
Integrase inhibitors (IIs)
Entry inhibitors (EIs): fusion inhibitors CCR5 inhibitors

Table 25.4 Contraception and HIV

Method	UKMEC category (no ART)	UKMEC category (using ART)
COC	1	2*
POP	1	2*
Progestogen-only injectables	1	1
Progestogen-only implants	1	2*
Cu-IUD	2	2
LNG-IUS	2	2
Condom	1	1
Diaphragms and caps	3	3

*Efficacy of the COC, POP and progestogen-only implant is affected by liver enzyme-inducing drugs, e.g. PIs and NNRTIs. Additional precautions are required. See individual chapters for recommendations.

Box 25.4 Side effects of ART

Hypersensitivity

Psychiatric problems

Lipodystrophy and lipoatrophy (characterized by redistribution of body fat)

Hyperlipidaemia

Abnormal liver or renal function

Peripheral neuropathy

Impaired glucose tolerance and diabetes (type 2)

Bone marrow suppression (anaemia, neutropenia)

Pancreatitis

Box 25.5 Strategies for HIV prevention

- Promoting safer sexual practices. Male condoms offer a high level of protection against HIV infection if used correctly and consistently. If used in sero-discordant couples the risk of HIV transmission is reduced by 80%
- HIV (and STI) testing and awareness
- Preventing mother-to-child transmission
- Male circumcision reduces the risk of heterosexually acquired HIV infection in men by ~60%
- Harm reduction for PWIDs, e.g. needle exchange programmes, prescription of substitutes
- Treatment as prevention (TASP): reduction of the viral load using ART reduces the likelihood of HIV transmission. This could be used in individual situations, e.g sero-discordant couples or on a larger scale
- PrEP – pre-exposure prophylaxis in specfic situations (Box 25.6)
- Provision of post-exposure prophylaxis (PEP & PEPSE, see Sexual Assault, Box 26.3)
- Screening blood and treating blood products

Box 25.6 Pre-exposure prophylaxis

- PrEP is daily use of ART by individuals who are HIV negative to prevent acquisition of infection

- Can be given systemically or topically (e.g. vaginal gel), on a daily basis

- RCTs have shown effectiveness in groups of participants

- Other trials are underway. Meantime use in the UK should be limited to the context of a clinical research study

- Unanswered questions include the impact on the emergence of drug resistance, toxicity of taking daily PrEP and the cost

- Avidity testing: measures the strength of antibody binding to viral proteins to give a guide to the recency of infection. A low avidity test is consistent with recent infection. Testing is not widely available. It can be useful in establishing a more accurate time frame for partner notification and is also useful for HIV surveillance
- Baseline testing at initial diagnosis of HIV infection should include HIV resistance testing, full blood count, and liver and renal function tests. An STI screen including testing for other BBVs should be offered

Screening (Boxes 25.2, 25.3, Table 25.2)

- Late diagnosis of HIV is associated with significant and avoidable morbidity and mortality
- Current UK Guidelines aim to increase the uptake of HIV testing and to encourage and normalize HIV testing in settings out with sexual health in order to reduce the levels of undiagnosed infection (currently 25%)
- Testing is recommended in all sexual health clinics, abortion services, drug dependency programmes and BBV services. It should also be considered in new patients registering in primary care and all routine medical admissions to hospital in regions with a local HIV prevalence of >2 in 1000
- Although a pre-test discussion is recommended, this does not need to be complex or prolonged. Its purpose is to establish valid verbal consent for the HIV test
- Repeat testing: annual testing is recommended for PWIDs and MSM should be offered a test every 6 months
- Testing can be used as an opportunity for risk reduction interventions, e.g. discussing safer sex, offering condoms, hepatitis B vaccination

Management

Management of individuals with HIV is complex and requires a multidisciplinary approach by appropriately trained specialists. The British HIV Association (BHIVA) has published standards of care for people living with HIV. Detailed management of HIV is out with the scope of this text. The decision about when to start antiretroviral treatment (ART) depends on several factors including HIV related symptoms, the CD4 count (preferably before ≤ 350 cells/μL), comorbidity and the presence of an AIDs diagnosis.

Antiretroviral therapy (ART)

ART is a combination of ARV medicines used to slow the rate of HIV replication. Highly active antiretroviral therapy (HAART) is the term used to describe a combination of anti-HIV drugs. HIV mutates as it replicates therefore a combination of drugs is used to avoid drug resistance. Compliance is also vital to minimize the likelihood of developing drug resistance.

HIV ART is a rapidly advancing field. ART is separated into different classes depending on the mechanism of action (Table 25.3). ART is associated with side effects. Common but minor side-effects include diarrhoea, nausea, fatigue, and skin rash. More serious side effects are listed in Box 25.4. Drug interactions can occur leading to both increased drug toxicity and decreased efficacy. PIs and NNRTIs are metabolized via the cytochrome p450 system and are most commonly affected. The following website gives accurate information about drug interactions: http://www.hiv-druginteractions.org

HIV and the law

- *Insurance and mortgages*: negative HIV tests should have no impact and do not need to be disclosed. A positive result will need to be disclosed however there are companies who will offer financial products to those living with HIV infection
- *Prosecution for transmitting HIV*: there have been several cases in the UK where HIV positive individuals have been successfully prosecuted for transmitting HIV to a sexual partner (some with a resulting custodial sentence). The law in Scotland differs from the rest of the UK in that conviction can occur even if transmission of HIV does not take place
- *Protection from discrimination*: there are equality laws protecting HIV positive individuals from discrimination

HIV and contraception (Table 25.4)

Provision of adequate contraceptive choice is important for the wellbeing of women living with HIV. Most contraceptive methods are suitable for women with HIV however special consideration should be made for women taking ART in view of potential interactions with hormonal contraceptive methods.

With typical use, male and female condoms may have high failure rates for contraception and therefore dual protection (i.e. use of condoms and another method) is the most effective way to prevent unintended pregnancy and reduce HIV transmission. Diaphragms and caps are conferred a UKMEC 3 as nonoxinol-9 increases the risk of HIV transmission. Male and female sterilization should also be considered if permanent contraception is required.

Pregnancy

- Vertical transmission of HIV is almost entirely preventable. Untreated, the mother to child transmission (MTCT) rate of HIV is approximately 25%. With interventions, this is reduced to <1%
- Universal HIV screening in antenatal services in the UK was introduced in 1999 and has been an extremely successful intervention with >96% uptake in testing. This has reduced the proportion of neonates at risk from HIV infection
- The aim of antenatal treatment with ART is to reduce the viral load (VL) to undetectable levels. If the viral load is <50 copies/mL at 36 weeks gestation then vaginal delivery can be offered. Pre-labour caesarean section (PLCS) should be considered in the presence of a higher viral load and also for women taking zidovudine monotherapy irrespective of the VL at time of delivery
- Infant post-exposure prophylaxis should be given and in developed countries. Breastfeeding should be avoided in HIV positive mothers

Strategies for prevention – Boxes 25.5, 25.6

Further resources

UK National Guidelines for HIV Testing 2008, British HIV Association, British Association of Sexual Health and HIV, British Infection Society. London http://www.bhiva.org/documents/guidelines/testing/glineshivtest08.pdf

Increasing the uptake of HIV testing among black Africans in England. NICE public health guidance 33 (2011). Available from www.nice.org.uk/guidance/PH33

British HIV Association. Standards of care for people living with HIV in 2012. London: British HIV Association; 2012.

British HIV Association. Management of HIV infection in pregnant women http://www.bhiva.org/documents/Guidelines/Treatment/2012/120430PregnancyGuidelines.pdf

26 Sexual assault

Box 26.1 Clinical history

- Date, time and location of the assault
- Details of the assailant(s) including gender, number, whether known to the complainant
- Whether the assailant has any known risk factors for BBVs
- Nature of the assault: vaginal/anal/oral, use of objects, condom use and if ejaculation occurred
- Menstrual history (LMP), current contraception, pre-and post-assault sexual history including date of last consensual sexual intercourse
- PMH, DH, allergies

Table 26.1 Timescales for DNA persistence

Nature of assault	Forensic timescale
Vaginal penetration	7 days
Oral penetration	2 days*
Anal penetration	3 days*
Digital penetration	12 hours*
Kissing, licking, biting	48 hours* or longer

*Timescales are the same for male and female complainants

Table 26.3 Investigations following sexual assault

At presentation:
- Blood samples: serum save (to be stored in the virus laboratory and can be tested at a later date if required)
- Baseline screen (NAAT) for chlamydia and gonorrhoea

14 days:
- Chlamydia/gonorrhoea/trichomonas testing

3 months:
- HIV, HBV, HCV, syphilis (or 4 months if started on PEPSE)

Box 26.2 Risk factors for HIV in sexual assault

- Assailant HIV positive
- Assailant from a high risk group (e.g. MSM, PWIDs)
- Background local HIV prevalence high*
- Type of assault: receptive anal intercourse
- Associated genital injuries
- Multiple assailants
- Multiple risk factors
- Repeated intercourse
- Complainant has current STI
- Defloration has occurred

* High prevalence area is > 1%

Table 26.2 Situations when post-exposure prophylaxis (PEPSE) for HIV is considered (reproduced from BASHH 2011)

Source HIV status	HIV positive viral load detectable or unknown	HIV positive viral load undetectable	Unknown HIV status from high prevalence group/area*	Unknown HIV status from low prevalence group/area
Receptive anal sex	Recommend	Recommend	Recommend	Not recommended
Insertive anal sex	Recommend	Not recommended	Consider†	Not recommended
Receptive vaginal sex	Recommend	Not recommended	Consider†	Not recommended
Insertive vaginal sex	Recommend	Not recommended	Consider†	Not recommended
Fellatio with ejaculation‡	Consider	Not recommended	Not recommended	Not recommended
Fellatio without ejaculation‡	Not recommended	Not recommended	Not recommended	Not recommended
Splash of semen into eye	Consider	Not recommended	Not recommended	Not recommended
Cunnilingus	Not recommended	Not recommended	Not recommended	Not recommended
Human bite§	Not recommended	Not recommended	Not recommended	Not recommended

* High prevalence groups within this recommendation are those where there is a significant likelihood of the source individual being HIV-positive. Within the UK at present, this is likely to be men who have sex with men and individuals who have immigrated to the UK from areas of high HIV prevalence (particularly sub-Saharan Africa).
† More detailed knowledge of local prevalence of HIV within communities may change these recommendations from consider to recommended in areas of particularly high HIV prevalence.
‡ PEP is not recommended for individuals receiving fellatio, i.e. inserting their penis into another's oral cavity.
§ A bite is assumed to constitute breakage of the skin with passage of blood.

Box 26.3 Preferred first-line HIV-PEPSE regimen

Truvada (contains tenofovir 245 mg and emtricitabine 200 mg) ONE tablet ONCE daily
plus
Raltegravir 400 mg (also called Isentress) ONE tablet, TWICE a day
} For 28 days

This regimen is also recommended for PEP, e.g. following occupational exposure to HIV

Box 26.4 Risk of HIV transmission

Risk of HIV transmission = risk that assailant is HIV positive
×
the risk of exposure

(Where risk of transmission is less than 1 in 10 000, PEPSE is not recommended)

Reference: UK guideline for the use of post-exposure prophylaxis for HIV following sexual exposure (2011).
British Association for Sexual Health and HIV, http://www.bashh.org/guidelines

Box 26.5 Antibiotic prophylaxis following sexual assault

Antibiotic prophylaxis (for chlamydia, gonorrhoea and trichomonas):

Ceftriaxone 500 mg i.m. stat
plus azithromycin 1 g orally stat
plus metronidazole 2 g orally stat

Source: Benn et al (2011), UK guidelines for the use of post-exposure prophylaxis for HIV following sexual exposure (2011), Table 4, p. 700. Reproduced with permission of SAGE Publications Ltd.

Sexual and Reproductive Health at a Glance, First Edition. Catriona Melville. © 2015 by John Wiley & Sons, Ltd. Published 2015 by John Wiley & Sons, Ltd.
Companion website: www.ataglanceseries.com/sexualhealth

Background

Sexual violence is a serious global public health and human rights issue with potentially serious short and long-term consequences for both physical and mental health. Sexual violence encompasses a wide spectrum ranging from the use of rape as a weapon of war to sexual assault taking place within longstanding relationships. Although women are the usual victims of sexual violence with a lifetime risk of up to 20%, men and children may also be affected.

Sexual assault disproportionately affects vulnerable women and is also linked with the consumption of alcohol. The majority of complainants know their assailant.

- *Legal definitions of sexual offences*: the laws governing sexual activity vary internationally and throughout the UK (see Fundamentals Box 1.4). Rape is defined as the non-consensual penetration of the vagina, mouth or anus by a penis (both sexes can be raped). By law penetration with an object other than a penis is not rape; however, other charges may be brought ('sexual assault by penetration'). The definition of consent is explicitly described in legal guidance. Child sex abuse is also encompassed in the legal frameworks
- *Services*: victims of sexual assault ('complainants') may present to a variety of services although often sexual assault is first reported to the police. A forensic examination can be carried out by the local police (clients are often seen in a Family Protection Unit – FPU) or increasingly in a Sexual Assault Referral Centre (SARC)
- *SARCs*: these are specialist medical and forensic services providing care for anyone who has been raped or sexually assaulted. Service users who are unsure or do not wish to report the assault to police at the time of the incident can have their forensic samples taken and stored, permitting them to decide at a later stage whether to proceed with police involvement. Most SARCs enable self referral as well as referral via the police

Management

Assess for serious injuries

Approximately half of people reporting sexual assault will have associated injuries (non-genital or genital). Individuals should be assessed and those with major trauma or serious injuries requiring urgent treatment should be referred to the appropriate services (i.e. A&E) without delay. Management of these injuries should take precedence over forensic examination. The absence of genital trauma does not imply consent.

History taking (Box 26.1)

A sensitive, non-judgemental approach and concise documentation is essential as the clinical notes may form part of the judicial process.

Police engagement

It is important to ascertain whether the complainant wishes to proceed with police engagement (reporting) at this stage. An alternative is 'third party reporting': the incident is reported to the local FPU without disclosing the complainant's details. Consent for this should still be obtained. In the UK fewer than 20% of individuals who have experienced sexual assault report it to the police. Reasons for non-engagement should be sensitively explored as the complainant may report the crime with appropriate support.

Forensic medical examination (FME)

- The purpose of the FME is to collect any physical evidence or specimens that may be used as evidence if criminal charges are laid. It is essential that FME is undertaken by appropriately trained staff in a forensically secure environment in order to avoid DNA contamination and preserve the chain of evidence. FME should be undertaken as soon as possible after the incident, however it can be carried out up to 7 days later depending on the nature of the assault. The timescales for persistence of DNA are summarized in Table 26.1
- The complainant should be advised not to eat, drink or brush their teeth; not to wash or bathe; to keep any sanitary wear and clothes (unwashed) and not to pass urine (important if there is suspicion of drug facilitated assault)
- The FME is usually documented on a proforma. All injuries are described and documented and samples are taken, e.g. genital fluid swabs
- Blood must be collected within 3 days and urine within 4 days in drug facilitated sexual assaults. Hair analysis can be undertaken after one month post-drug ingestion if presentation is delayed
- Early evidence kits are available in some services and police forces. They contain a urine sample pot, mouth swab and mouth rinse to enable early collection of DNA evidence and toxicology

Immediate care

- *HIV post-exposure prophylaxis after sexual exposure (HIV PEPSE)*: a case-by-case risk assessment should be undertaken (Table 26.2 and Boxes 26.2–26.4). If indicated, PEPSE should be commenced as soon as possible and no later than 72 hours after the assault. A baseline HIV test should be taken before starting PEPSE. Studies have demonstrated that PEPSE can reduce the risk of HIV acquisition by about 80% after sexual assault if given early and continued for 28 days
- *HBV PEP*: if not already vaccinated, this can be commenced up to 6 weeks post assault. An accelerated schedule should be followed. HBV immunoglobulin can also be considered preferably within 48 hours but up to 7 days following a single high risk exposure in a non-immune individual (see Chapter 24)
- *Emergency contraception (EC)*: a pregnancy risk assessment should be undertaken and either hormonal EC or a CU-IUD offered if appropriate (see Chapter 7)
- *STI testing and prophylaxis (Table 26.3 and Box 26.5)*: baseline STI testing can be offered, however a further test will need to undertaken 14 days after the assault. Non-invasive or self-taken swabs can be offered for individuals who do not require or decline a speculum examination. Sites for sampling should be determined from the history. The advantages versus the disadvantages of antibiotic prophylaxis for STIs should be considered i.e. missed opportunity for PN, versus individual likely to default from follow-up

Psychological consequences

- Anxiety and depression are common after sexual assault. The minority of individuals may go on to develop post-traumatic stress disorder (PTSD). Individuals should be referred to appropriate services and given information about local victim support organizations e.g. rape crisis

Follow-up

- Appointments should be arranged for repeat STI and BBV testing out with the window period and for completion of the HBV vaccination schedule. The need for ongoing psychosocial support should be evaluated at follow up

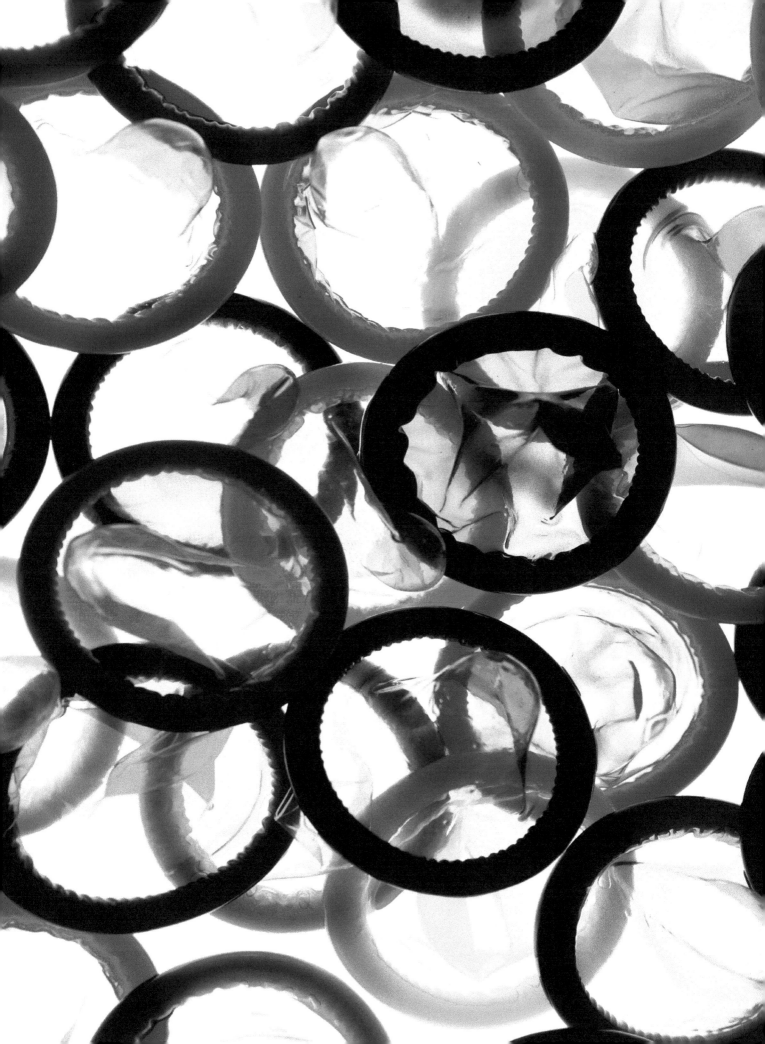

Reproductive health

 Don't forget to visit the companion website at www.ataglanceseries.com/sexualhealth where you can test yourself on these topics.

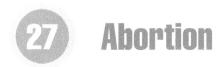

27 Abortion

Box 27.1 Grounds for abortion in Great Britain

Two registered medical practitioners must agree that the pregnancy should be terminated on one or more of the following grounds:

A The continuance of the pregnancy would involve risk to the life of the pregnant woman greater than if the pregnancy were terminated

B The termination is necessary to prevent grave permanent injury to the physical or mental health of the pregnant woman

C The pregnancy has not exceeded its 24th week and that the continuance of the pregnancy would involve risk, greater than if the pregnancy were terminated, of injury to the physical or mental health of the pregnant woman

D The pregnancy has not exceeded its 24th week and that the continuance of the pregnancy would involve risk, greater than if the pregnancy were terminated, of injury to the physical or mental health of any existing children of the family of the pregnant woman

E There is a substantial risk that if the child were born it would suffer from such physical or mental abnormalities as to be seriously handicapped

In an emergency, authorization can be by a single doctor who is undertaking the procedure:

F To save the life of the pregnant woman

G To prevent grave permanent injury to the physical or mental health of the pregnant woman

Table 27.1 Pre-abortion investigations

Blood tests
- Determination of rhesus status (essential)
- Determination of blood group with screening for red cell antibodies ⎤
- Haemoglobin concentration   → Only where clinically indicated
- Testing for haemoglobinopathies ⎦
- HIV and syphilis (see STI screening)

VTE risk assessment
- Is recommended in NICE Clinical Guideline 92

Cervical cytology screening
- Offer or arrange screening if missed or overdue

Ultrasound scan – *see notes*
- To determine gestation
- To exclude ectopic pregnancy

STI screening – *see notes*
- *C. trachomatis* (recommended) ⎤
- *Neisseria gonorrhoeae* (depending on   → e.g. by self-taken
  risk assessment and local prevalence) ⎦ vulvovaginal swab
- HIV (recommended: UK National Guidelines for HIV Testing 2008, BHIVA, BASHH, BIS)
- Syphilis (depending on risk assessment)

Box 27.2 Causes of unintended pregnancy

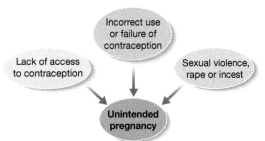

Incorrect use or failure of contraception

Lack of access to contraception

Sexual violence, rape or incest

Unintended pregnancy

Box 27.3 Options for women with an unintended pregnancy

Options

Continue with the pregnancy with additional support if required and keep the baby

Continue with the pregnancy and place the baby for adoption

End the pregnancy by having an abortion

Background

What is it? Induced abortion (sometimes known as termination of pregnancy – TOP) is a procedure undertaken to intentionally end a pregnancy by expulsion or removal of the fetus. This chapter will focus on induced abortion undertaken for reasons other than fetal anomaly. Abortion is one of the most commonly undertaken gynaecological procedures.

Global overview: The estimated absolute number of abortions worldwide in 2008 was 43.8 million, although obtaining accurate global abortion data is difficult as procedures are often under reported in countries where restrictive laws apply and even in liberal countries data must be retrieved from multiple sources. The subject of abortion often courts controversy and ethical and political debate. Although abortion is legal in the majority of countries including the UK, it is still outlawed or severely restricted in many regions worldwide. Restricting or banning abortion does not reduce the abortion rate in these countries, but instead women may seek this procedure from illegal and unsafe providers; self-induce abortion; or be forced to travel to a different country (with more liberal laws) to access a service. It is estimated that there are 47,000 deaths worldwide each year from unsafe abortion. Most of these occur in developing countries. In contrast, legal abortion performed by competent individuals in sterile facilities is a safe procedure with a low incidence of morbidity and mortality.

Legal issues

Most countries will allow abortion to save a women's life, although the uncertainty professionals face in some countries when determining who meets this criteria were illustrated in a high profile case in The Republic of Ireland in 2012:

Savita Halappanavar

This 31 year-old woman was admitted to a hospital in the Republic of Ireland in 2012, suffering from an inevitable miscarriage at 17 weeks gestation. Her condition worsened and she developed sepsis, however the welfare of her unborn (and non-viable) fetus was prioritised over her health during the following 3 days and she subsequently died of septic shock. An investigation into her death concluded that uncertainty relating to the law on abortion in Ireland contributed to her death. Doctors were fearful to act in case criminal proceedings were brought against them should they have aborted the fetus to save the mother's life.

As a consequence, new abortion legislation was introduced in Ireland in 2013. In the USA and Australia abortion is legal however each state or territory will have its own laws governing the procedure. In other countries such as Malta and many parts of Latin America abortion is criminalized in most circumstances.

In Great Britain (England, Scotland and Wales but not Northern Ireland) abortion is governed by the Abortion Act 1967 (amended in 1990 by the Human Fertilisation and Embryology Act) which allows abortion up to 24 weeks' gestation if certain criteria are met (Box 27.1), and abortion over 24 weeks' gestation in exceptional circumstances (e.g. to save the woman's life, or for severe fetal anomalies). Any treatment for the termination of pregnancy can only be carried out in an NHS hospital or in a place approved for the purpose by the Secretary of State, and after 24 weeks, only in an NHS hospital (except in an emergency).

The majority of abortions in Britain (over 95%) are undertaken under Ground C. In Britain prior to an abortion, two doctors must complete a'"Grounds for carrying out an abortion' form (e.g. HSA1 in England or Certificate A in Scotland), and following the procedure an'"Abortion Notification form' must be sent to the Chief Medical Officer (CMO).

Although part of the United Kingdom, the Abortion Act of 1967 does not extend to Northern Ireland, where abortions are governed by the Offences Against the Person Act 1861. This Act effectively outlaws abortion in all but exceptional cases. On average five women a day travel from Northern Ireland to mainland Britain to obtain an abortion (at their own expense).

Role of health care professionals

- **Doctors** are responsible for completing the legal documents, prescribing any drugs required for the procedure and taking overall responsibility for the abortion process in Great Britain and most other countries
- **Nurses and midwives** can administer the drugs required for an abortion at any gestation once they have been prescribed by a doctor, but in Britain, and the majority of developed countries they cannot perform surgical abortions. There is growing support however to expand the role of mid-level health care providers (nurse practitioners, midwives, physicians assistants, etc.) in abortion care. In South Africa nurse practitioners and physicians assistants have been able to provide first-trimester abortion services since 1997. More recently (2013), the state of California in the USA passed legislation to allow trained mid-level healthcare workers to provide first trimester aspiration abortions. As evidence grows that abortion is safe when undertaken by these competent providers, their role is likely to expand in many countries

Conscientious objection

- The Abortion Act contains a conscientious objection clause
- Health practitioners can refuse to participate in abortion treatment if it conflicts with their moral or religious beliefs
- Doctors who have a conscientious objection to abortion must tell women of their right to see another doctor
- This clause does not apply when treatment is required in an emergency situation, e.g. to save life or prevent grave permanent injury to the woman's physical or mental healt

Referral and service providers

Referral

Women often seek advice and referral from their primary care provider (GP or practice nurse) or community reproductive health clinic in the event of an unplanned pregnancy. Alternatively, some abortion services will accept self-referrals. Many abortion providers have close links with other services, e.g. addictions services or the Looked After Accommodated Children (LAAC) team to allow swift access to the service and minimize delays, particularly in the most vulnerable groups of women. National standards exist regarding referral timeframes for abortion. The RCOG recommends that women are offered an assessment appointment within 5 working days of referral as the earlier in pregnancy an abortion is performed the safer it is.

Box 27.4 Medical abortion drugs

Antiprogesterone (Mifepristone)
A synthetic steroid and progesterone receptor antagonist. Binds to progesterone receptors, inhibiting the action of progesterone thus interfering with the continuation of the pregnancy. It increases the sensitivity of the uterus to prostaglandins. Used in conjunction with prostaglandins for medical abortion at all gestations.
Dose: 200 mg, orally

Prostaglandin (e.g. misoprostol, gemeprost)
A synthetic prostaglandin analogue; enhances uterine contractions and aids expulsion of products of conception.
Dose: misoprostol 400–800 μg depending on gestation. Can be administered vaginally, sublingually, buccally or orally

Table 27.2 Types of procedures at different gestations

Pregnancy gestation (weeks)	Medical methods	Surgical methods	
4	**Early medical abortion ≤ 63 days**	**< 49 days**	
5	• Single oral dose of Mifepristone, e.g. 200 mg followed 24 – 48 hours later by:	Early vacuum aspiration (EVA)	
6			
7	• Single dose of prostaglandin, e.g. misoprostol 800 μg (vaginal, buccal or sublingual routes)		
8		**7 – 14 weeks**	
9		Electric or manual vacuum aspiration (EVA or MVA)	
10			
11			
12			
13	**Medical abortion at 64 days – 24 weeks**		
14	• Single oral dose of Mifepristone e.g. 200 mg followed 36 – 48 hours later by:	**14 – 16 weeks**	
15		Vacuum aspiration with large-bore (15.9 mm diameter) cannula and suction tube	
16	• Multiple doses of prostaglandin e.g. misoprostol 800 μg (vaginal, buccal or sublingual routes) then 3-hourly doses of misoprostol 400 μg (to a maximum of four further doses)		
17			
18			
19			**15 – 24 weeks**
20			Dilatation and evacuation (D&E)
21			
22			
23			
24			

Box 27.5 Cervical priming before surgical abortion

1 Prostaglandin analogues

• Recommended up to 14 weeks' gestation
• Misoprostol 400 μg vaginally 3 hours prior to surgery (women can self-administer) or sublingually 2 – 3 hours prior to surgery
• Can be used between 14 – 18 weeks' gestation but osmotic dilators are more effective

2 Osmotic dilators

• Absorbent rods inserted into the cervix, which absorb fluid from the surrounding tissues and swell causing gentle cervical dilatation
• Superior to prostaglandins after 14 weeks' gestation
• Require at least 4 hours in situ to be effective but often inserted overnight before D&E

Figure 27.1 Vacuum aspiration techniques

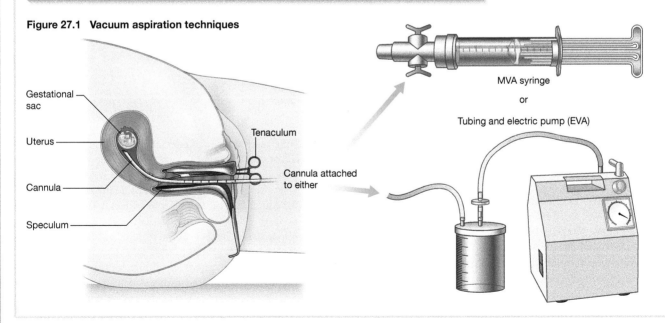

Gestational sac
Uterus
Cannula
Speculum
Tenaculum
Cannula attached to either
MVA syringe
or
Tubing and electric pump (EVA)

Abortion providers

Abortions may be provided within the public sector (e.g. NHS), or by independent or charitable organizations. These services may fall within the remit of hospital gynaecology departments although increasingly community based SRH services are responsible for providing abortion. The type and location of abortion services is largely determined by the country in which the service is located and its governing legislation. In Scotland, 98% of abortions are provided within the public sector (NHS), whereas in England although 97% of procedures are funded by the NHS, only 35% of these are undertaken in NHS hospitals, the remainder being undertaken in the independent sector, e.g. Marie Stopes International (MSI) or British Pregnancy Advisory Service (BPAS). An alternative to attending a service is to access medical abortion via a web-based service. Women on Web (WoW) enables women to access a medical consultation via an interactive web-based questionnaire and to receive the drugs required for medical abortion via postal mail. In countries where abortion is illegal or highly restricted, or the drugs for medical abortion are not available, this service can offer an alternative to unsafe abortion.

Pre-abortion assessment

Pre-abortion discussion: Not all women considering an abortion have an unplanned or even unwanted pregnancy. Changes in a women's health or socioeconomic circumstances can result in women seeking an abortion for a planned and much wanted pregnancy. Some reasons for women seeking an abortion are listed in Box 27.2. Equally, not all women attending an assessment clinic will decide on an abortion and it is important to discuss all the available choices during this initial consultation in a non-directional manner, including offering support which may be appropriate (e.g. department of social work). This will enable the woman to make an informed decision. There are three main options available to women with an unintended pregnancy (Box 27.3). Women may need time to consider these options before making a decision or may choose to access more formal counselling services. This should be facilitated in a timely manner.

Pre-abortion counselling: In some countries counselling is mandatory prior to having an abortion. An example is Texas in the USA, where from late 2013, women must receive state-directed counselling that includes information designed to discourage proceeding with an abortion and then wait 24 hours before the procedure is provided. The introduction of mandatory independent counselling in the UK was also debated recently but has not been introduced. Many view these developments as impeding access to safe and timely abortion access for women.

Investigations: Table 27.1 lists the investigations to be considered before an abortion. Most women will undergo an ultrasound scan as part of their initial assessment; however RCOG guidance does not recommend this as a prerequisite to abortion although there should be access to it if required. Provision of STI screening varies by service. A risk assessment and consideration of the local prevalence of STI's such as gonorrhoea is useful when planning abortion service protocols.

Contraception: Future contraception should be discussed before the procedure and a plan made for commencing the chosen method post-abortion.

Abortion procedures

Abortion may be undertaken using medical or surgical methods at all gestations up to 24 weeks. The choice of method will depend on patient preference, local availability and the gestation of the pregnancy. Some techniques are more appropriate at different gestation bands (Table 27.2).

Medical abortion

Since medical methods of abortion were licensed for use in the UK in 1991, an increasing number of abortions are being performed medically. The proportion of medical abortions trebled in the last decade in England and Wales, and in 2013, over 78% of procedures were performed medically in Scotland.

Drug information

Medical abortion employs the use of 2 drugs (Box 27.4); an antiprogesterone (mifepristone), followed 24–72 hours (usually 48 hours) later by a prostaglandin (e.g. misoprostol). In the UK the prostaglandin gemeprost is licensed for abortion procedures however it is expensive and requires storage below minus 10°C, so conventionally misoprostol is used although this is out with product licence. Many of the medical regimens used for abortion are unlicensed for such use however these drugs can be used out with licence in the UK as long as the woman is aware that it is being used for an unlicensed indication.

Route of administration

Misoprostol can be administered orally, vaginally, sublingually or bucally; however, after 49 days, vaginal misoprostol is more effective than the oral route. Sublingual or buccal routes of misoprostol administration are associated with more adverse effects than vaginal routes (e.g. headache) and are associated with an unpleasant taste in the mouth.

Place of abortion

Although the medication for abortion must be administered in licensed premises in Great Britain, there is no restriction on where the actual abortion takes place. Many services now offer early discharge home for abortions at gestations up to 63 days. The woman leaves the hospital following administration of misoprostol and completes the procedure at home. Adequate support and rigorous follow-up arrangements must be made for these women.

Surgical abortion

Vacuum aspiration can be performed up to 16 weeks' gestation with the following caveats:

- Below 7 weeks the failure rate is higher than at later gestations and a rigorous protocol should be followed including inspection of the aspirated tissue and further evaluation (e.g. serum βHCG) if the products are not identified
- Between 14 and 16 weeks large bore cannulae must be used, which may not be readily available in Great Britain. Only experienced clinicians should be undertaking procedures at this gestation
- **Cervical preparation** should be considered in all women undergoing surgical abortion to reduce the risk of uterine perforation or cervical trauma (Box 27.5)

Vacuum aspiration involves evacuation of the uterus using a cannula attached to a vacuum source. The vacuum is either generated using an electrical (EVA) or manual source (MVA) (Figure 27.1).

Figure 27.2 Double-valve MVA syringe

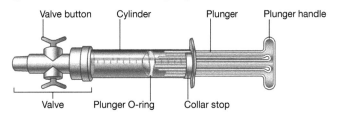

Valve button Cylinder Plunger Plunger handle

Valve Plunger O-ring Collar stop

Figure 27.3 MVA cannula

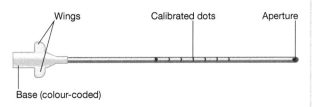

Wings Calibrated dots Aperture

Base (colour-coded)

Table 27.3 Abortion complications

Complication	Method	
	Medical abortion	**Surgical abortion**
Failed abortion	Both procedures carry a small risk of failure to end the pregnancy of less than 1 in 100	
Haemorrhage (severe bleeding requiring blood transfusion)	Increases with increasing gestation: • Less than 1 in 1000 for early abortions • About 4 in 1000 for abortions > 20 weeks gestation	
Incomplete abortion (RPOC†) requiring intervention	Usually much less than 5% of women will require further intervention, e.g. evacuation of RPOC after medical abortion	
Uterine perforation	N/A	1 – 4 in 1000 (risk reduces with earlier gestation and with experience of clinician)
Cervical trauma (damage to the external cervical os)	N/A	1 in 100 (risk reduces with earlier gestation and with experience of clinician)
Uterine rupture	Less than 1 in 1000 (midtrimester* abortions only)	N/A
Post-abortion infection	See Box 27.6	

*Midtrimester abortions = 13 – 24 weeks
†RPOC = retained products of conception

Box 27.7 Post-abortion care

• Anti-D IgG 250 IU should be administered to all non-sensitized RhD-negative women within 72 hours of abortion (medical or surgical)

• Women should be advised of symptoms they may experience which would warrant seeking medical attention

• Routine follow-up is unnecessary if successful abortion has been confirmed at the time of the procedure

• Contraception should be provided immediately after abortion. Women should be informed of the greater effectiveness of the LARC methods

• Post-abortion counselling should be available to women who request this

Box 27.6 Prevention of infective sequelae

Pelvic infection will occur in up to 10% of women undergoing abortion if there is no intervention

Interventions include:
• Prophylaxis for all (minimum standard)
• Screen all women and treat only those who test positive ('screen and treat')
• Screen all women and give prophylaxis to all women

Prophylactic antibiotic regimen example:
• Azithromycin 1 g orally
plus
• Metronidazole 1 g rectally

Note:
Partner notification should be undertaken or arranged for women who test positive for an STI

Figure 27.4 Local anaesthesia

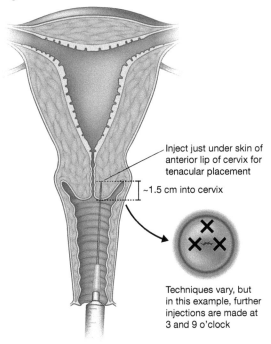

Inject just under skin of anterior lip of cervix for tenacular placement

~1.5 cm into cervix

Techniques vary, but in this example, further injections are made at 3 and 9 o'clock

MVA employs a hand-held syringe or aspirator which is connected to a cannula and used to create a vacuum manually (Figures 27.2, 27.3). This technique is growing in popularity in Great Britain. It is often performed with a local anaesthetic, and safety, efficacy and levels of satisfaction are similar to EVA. Surgeons report more procedural difficulties using MVA over 9 weeks' gestation, so for this reason many services offer EVA at later gestations. The maximum cannula diameter available for MVA is 12 mm.

Feticide

To negate the risk of a live birth, feticide (e.g. via ultrasound guided intracardiac potassium chloride injection) should be performed before medical abortion after 21 weeks 6 days' gestation.

Analgesia and anaesthesia

Surgical abortion can be performed under local (para- or intracervical) anaesthetic, conscious sedation or general anaesthetic. Intracervical block has less risk of vascular injection than paracervical block and is safe and effective (Figure 27.4). MVA is traditionally performed under local anaesthetic whereas EVA often employs general anaesthesia in Great Britain. Analgesia is routinely offered during both medical and surgical abortion e.g. non-steroidal anti-inflammatory drugs (NSAIDs). Medical abortion at later gestations may require the use of narcotic analgesia.

Risks, complications and adverse effects

Overall abortion is a safe procedure with a low risk of major complications and extremely low risk of mortality in the UK (Table 27.3). The risks increase with increasing gestation hence the importance of early access and minimising the delays to abortion services.

- **Post-abortion infection:** there are several strategies used to prevent complications from infection (Box 27.6). Screening is important as it provides an opportunity to treat the partner of an infected woman thus preventing re-infection. Peri-abortion antibiotic prophylaxis should be provided for women undergoing medical or surgical abortion and should utilize drugs which are effective against *C. trachomatis* and anaerobes (Box 27.6)
- **Breast cancer:** there is no association between abortion and an increase in breast cancer risk
- **Future reproductive outcomes**: abortion is not associated with subsequent infertility, placenta praevia or ectopic pregnancy however there is some evidence to suggest an association with a small increased risk of future preterm delivery. The evidence is insufficient to demonstrate causality
- **Psychological sequelae:** women may experience a range of emotions around the time of an unplanned pregnancy. Those with pre-existing mental health problems may experience further problems whether they continue with the pregnancy or have an abortion. There is no evidence that proceeding with an abortion negatively impacts on psychological wellbeing any more than continuing with the pregnancy and having the baby

Disposal of fetal tissue

Fetal tissue should be disposed of with sensitivity and dignity in accordance with National legislation and local policy. Recent guidance from the Scottish Government advises that a minimum standard is collective disposal of pregnancy tissue in a crematorium. Women should be informed of the options available for fetal disposal and their wishes met wherever possible Options generally include cremation or burial, but women can make their own arrangements. Conversely, some women do not wish to participate in a detailed dialogue regarding disposal of fetal tissue and this decision should also be respected.

Post-abortion care and follow-up

A summary is provided in Box 27.7. Although routine follow-up after abortion is not required, a review to exclude a continuing pregnancy may be required with medical abortion, particularly if this has taken place at home and there is uncertainty as to whether the products of conception (POC) have passed. Confirmation may be by means of a follow-up ultrasound scan, or alternatively by urine HCG testing (patient self-testing at home) with telephone review.

Contraception

Immediate provision of all methods of contraception should be available in abortion services. The efficacy of the LARC methods should be emphasized. Ideally all methods should be initiated on the day of the surgical procedure or the second part of the medical procedure. In this instance, the methods will be immediately effective. If the POP, a combined hormonal method, progestogen only injection or implant are initiated more than 5 days after the abortion, then additional precautions will be required (e.g. barrier methods or abstinence). The starting regimens for each method are detailed in the relevant chapters. There is an increased incidence of regret if sterilization is undertaken at the time of an abortion therefore it is advisable to delay this procedure for at least 6 weeks. In order to avoid a further unplanned pregnancy during this time, consideration should be given to provision of a bridging method of contraception until the time of the procedure. It is suggested that an intrauterine method (Cu-IUD or LNG-IUS) is inserted at the time of surgical abortion or immediately following the second part of medical abortion or within 48 hours of these procedures. Otherwise, practice has been to delay insertion for a further 4 weeks. There is not however any evidence that insertion of an intrauterine device between 48 hours and 4 weeks post abortion increases the risk of perforation and it can be undertaken by an experienced clinician once the procedure has been confirmed complete. Again, if there is any delay initiating one of these methods, a bridging method should be initiated in the interim.

Useful resources

The Care of Women Requesting Induced Abortion. RCOG Evidence Based Clinical Guideline Number 7. November 2011 https://www.rcog.org.uk/en/guidelines-research-services/guidelines/the-care-of-women-requesting-induced-abortion/

British Pregnancy Advisory Service (BPAS) www.bpas.org

Marie Stopes International http://www.mariestopes.org/

International Pregnancy Advisory Service (IPAS) www.ipas.org (has step by step MVA guide)

28 Abnormal uterine bleeding

Table 28.1 AUB terminology

Abnormal uterine bleeding (AUB)	Abnormal uterine bleeding (AUB) is any menstrual bleeding from the uterus that is either abnormal in volume, regularity and timing or is non-menstrual (IMB, PCB, PMB)
Heavy menstrual bleeding (HMB)	Excessive menstrual blood loss (MBL) which interferes with the woman's physical, emotional, social and material quality of life
Post-coital bleeding (PCB)	Non-menstrual genital tract bleeding immediately after (or shortly after) intercourse
Intermenstrual bleeding (IMB)	Uterine bleeding occurring between predictable and clearly defined cyclic menses
Breakthrough bleeding (BTB)	Unscheduled bleeding in women using hormonal contraception
Post-menopausal bleeding (PMB)	Bleeding from the genital tract occurring 1 year after the menopause (LMP)

Table 28.2 PALM–COEIN classification of AUB

Polyp (endometrial, cervical)	Coagulopathy
Adenomyosis	Ovulatory dysfunction e.g. PCOS
Leiomyoma → submucosal or other	Endometrial
Malignancy (of the genital tract) and hyperplasia	Iatrogenic, e.g. CU-IUD
	Not yet classified

Box 28.1 Causes of HMB

- No cause found: 40 – 60%
- Uterine fibroids 20 – 30%
- Uterine polyps 5 – 10%
- Adenomyosis 5%
- Endometriosis < 5%
- Endometrial hyperplasia or malignancy (usually presents with IMB, PCB or PMB)
- Pelvic inflammatory disease or infection
- Hypothyroidism
- Coagulation disorders (e.g. von Willebrand disease)
- Iatrogenic: anti-coagulants, Cu-IUD

Figure 28.1 Endometrial biopsy

Indications	• Persistent IMB • Age ≥ 45 years • Treatment failure or ineffective treatment
Procedure	Blind endometrial biopsy can be taken using a fine-bore plastic instrument, e.g. the Pipelle. It has a central plunger which creates a vacuum when pulled. It is tolerated well, usually without local anaesthesia and has similar sensitivity to D&C for detecting endometrial cancer and hyperplasia

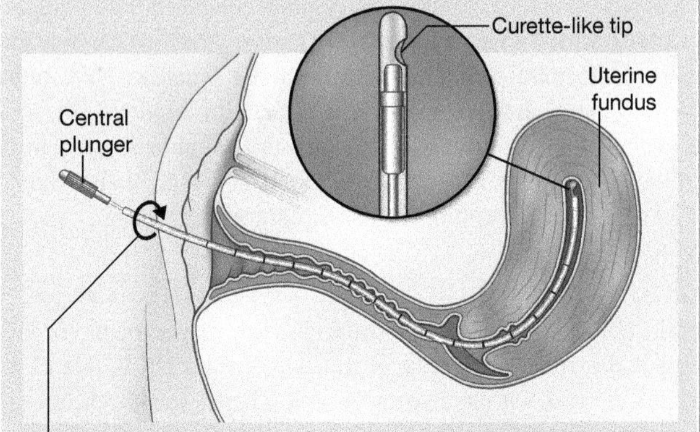

Curette-like tip

Uterine fundus

Central plunger

Instrument rotated slowly once plunger pulled back and removed slowly

Sample of endometrium removed by suction

Box 28.2 Risk factors for endometrial hyperplasia and cancer

- Obesity
- PCOS
- Diabetes
- Tamoxifen
- Unopposed oestrogen therapy
- Family history of endometrial cancer
- Hypertension
- Nulliparity
- Perimenopausal and postmenopausal age groups

Abnormal uterine bleeding (AUB) (Table 28.1)

Abnormal uterine bleeding (AUB) is any menstrual bleeding from the uterus that is either abnormal in volume, regularity and timing or is non-menstrual (IMB, PCB, PMB).

- Classification: the PALM-COEIN classification system for AUB was approved by FIGO in 2011 (Table 28.2)

Heavy menstrual bleeding (HMB)

- Prevalence: HMB is extremely common affecting 3% of premenopausal women and accounting for almost 15% of gynaecological referrals in the UK
- Aetiology (Box 28.1): 40–60% of women with HMB have no uterine, endocrine, haematological or infective pathology on investigation (formerly termed as having dysfunctional uterine bleeding – DUB). Their symptoms are probably due to a combination of ovulatory or endometrial dysfunction or coagulopathy

Assessment

- In all woman of reproductive age, pregnancy should be excluded
- **History**: objective measurement of MBL does not influence management and in clinical practice, subjective measurement is used (clinical history); determine the nature of the bleeding, i.e. frequency, duration, volume (clots, flooding, sanitary protection), cycle regularity. Enquire about associated symptoms of pelvic pain or pressure effects (gastrointestinal or genitourinary). Check the cervical screening history
- If the history suggests HMB without structural or histological abnormality then first-line treatment can be commenced without the need for further examination or investigations (unless inserting an LNG-IUS)
- A history of PCB, PMB, IMB, pelvic pain, dyspareunia, pelvic mass or pressure symptoms (bowel or bladder) may be suggestive of pathology, e.g. fibroids, malignancy or endometriosis

Examination

Abdominal and bimanual pelvic examination should be undertaken if pathology is suspected; prior to LNG-IUS insertion; or if there is treatment failure. The finding of an enlarged uterus or cervical lesion requires further investigation or referral as appropriate.

Investigations

- Full blood count should be taken in all women presenting with HMB
- A cervical smear should be taken only if screening is due
- A coagulation screen should only be taken if indicated by the personal or family history
- An STI screen if indicated by the history (can be taken by non-invasive testing if examination not indicated)
- Endometrial biopsy (Figure 28.1)
- Imaging should be arranged if the uterus is palpable abdominally, or there is a pelvic mass on vaginal examination or medical treatment fails. Ultrasound is the first-line imaging tool. If ultrasound is inconclusive then hysteroscopy can be undertaken

Management

Pharmaceutical treatment

- First-line: LNG-IUS
- Second line: tranexamic acid or NSAIDs (e.g. mefenamic acid, ibuprofen) or COC
- Progestogens: oral norethisterone (15 mg) daily (days 5–26) or DMPA 12 weekly by IM injection

Surgical treatments

- Endometrial ablation, e.g. thermal balloon/microwave ablation. Future pregnancy must be avoided after ablation
- Myomectomy or uterine artery embolization for fibroids
- Hysterectomy: should not be first line treatment solely for HMB

Unscheduled bleeding on hormonal contraception

- Before starting hormonal contraception women should be informed of the likely bleeding patterns associated with the method of choice (see contraceptive chapters). Unscheduled bleeding is common in the first 3–6 months of hormonal contraceptive use. It is more common with progestogen-only than combined methods
- Aetiology: the exact mechanism of unscheduled bleeding with hormonal contraceptives is unknown. Other pathologies, e.g. STIs, cervical polyp or ectopy may be responsible. Cervical cancer is rare, particularly if the screening programme has been adhered to. Endometrial malignancy is also rare in women of reproductive age, unless there are additional risk factors (Box 28.2)
- **History**: the cervical screening history should be confirmed, and risk factors for pregnancy and STIs explored. Ask about other medication (possible drug interactions) and any associated symptoms (e.g. pelvic pain, PCB). Verify compliance with the method (e.g. no missed pills)
- **Examination:** in first 3 months of method use, examination is not required if cervical screening is current and there are no coexistent symptoms. If bleeding persists beyond 3 months, cervical screening is due or at the request of the woman, an examination should be undertaken. (speculum ± bimanual)
- **Investigations**: are dictated by the clinical findings and may include a pregnancy test, cervical smear, STI screen, endometrial biopsy and ultrasound scan
- **Management**: options are fairly limited. Persisting with the method chosen rather than swapping within the first few months is advised as bleeding patterns may settle. For treatment of women using progestogen-only methods the COC may be used for up to 3 months either continuously or cyclically (out with license). Once reassured that there is no underlying pathology, some individuals may choose to continue using the method as the advantages may outweigh the disadvantages

Postcoital bleeding (PCB)

- Aetiology: Cervical polyp, cervical ectopy, STI (e.g. chlamydia, gonorrhoea), cervical intraepithelial neoplasia (CIN) or invasive cervical cancer (uncommon). No specific cause is found in about 50% of women with PCB

Intermenstrual bleeding (IMB)

- Aetiology: endometrial polyps, fibroids, inflammatory response with Cu-IUD, endometritis due to an STI
- Assessment of PCB and IMB is the same as with other bleeding problems (as above)

References

Munro MG, Critchley HO, Broder MS, Fraser IS and the FIGO Working Group on Menstrual Disorders. FIGO classification system (PALM-COEIN) for causes of abnormal uterine bleeding in nongravid women of reproductive age. *Int J Gynaecol Obstet* 2011;113:3–13

National Institute for Health and Care Excellence. Heavy menstrual bleeding, Clinical Guideline 44. London: NICE; 2007. www.nice.org.uk/CG44

Faculty of Sexual and Reproductive Healthcare clinical guidance. Management of Unscheduled Bleeding in Women using Hormonal Contraception. FSRH 2009. www.fsrh.org/pdfs/UnscheduledBleedingMay09.pdf

29 Menstrual problems

Table 29.1 Causes of primary amenorrhoea

Physiological	Pregnancy Constitutional delay: a common cause, no anatomical abnormality, frequently familial, diagnosis by exclusion of pathology
Pathological	Hypothalamic: chronic systemic illness, weight loss, exercise, stress, depression Genitourinary malformations: imperforate hymen, transverse septum, absent vagina or uterus, Meyer–Rokinstansky–Kustner–Hauser syndrome Genetic: androgen insensitivity syndrome, Turners syndrome, late onset congenital adrenal hyperplasia Pituitary: prolactinoma Iatrogenic: (medications) chemotherapy, radiotherapy, antipsychotic drugs

Table 29.2 Causes of oligomenorrhoea and secondary amenorrhoea

Physiological	Pregnancy, lactation, menopause
Hypothalamic	Chronic systemic illness, weight loss, eating disorders, exercise, stress, depression
Pituitary	Prolactinoma, head injury, Sheehan's syndrome (pituitary infarction after major obstetric haemorrhage), hyperprolactinaemia (stress, drugs)
Ovarian	Premature ovarian failure, PCOS
Endocrine	Thyroid disorders, Cushing's syndrome
Uterine	Asherman's syndrome (intrauterine adhesions), cervical stenosis
Chromosomal	Fragile X, mosaic Turner's syndrome
Iatrogenic/illicit drugs	Chemotherapy, radiotherapy, antipsychotic drugs, cocaine, opiates

Box 29.1 Treatment of dysmenorrhoea

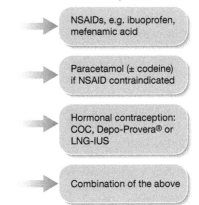

- NSAIDs, e.g. ibuoprofen, mefenamic acid
- Paracetamol (± codeine) if NSAID contraindicated
- Hormonal contraception: COC, Depo-Provera® or LNG-IUS
- Combination of the above

Table 29.3 Investigations for oligomenorrhoea and amenorrhoea

LH, FSH (taken during menses if oligomenorrhoea)	•High FSH levels (> 20 IU/L on two occasions) suggests premature ovarian failure •Low or normal FSH levels are found with weight loss, stress and excessive exercise (suggests a hypothalamic problem) •Increased LH/FSH ratio found with PCOS (LH > 10 IU/L)
Testosterone	> 5 nmol/L suggests androgen-secreting tumour or Cushing's syndrome. Refer to specialist
Prolactin	> 1000 mIU/L suggests pituitary adenoma (normal is < 500 mIU/L). Refer to specialist
TSH	High TSH indicates hypothyroidism. Refer to specialist

Figure 29.1 Rotterdam diagnostic criteria for PCOS

PCOS can be diagnosed if 2 out of 3 of the following criteria are present (and other causes of hyperandrogenism are excluded):

- Amenorrhoea or oligomenorrhoea

- Clinical and/or biochemical evidence of excess androgens (and exclusion of other ætiologies)

- Polycystic ovaries: large volume ovaries (> 10 cm³) and/or multiple small follicles (12 or more follicles < 10 mm)

Reference: The Rotterdam ESHRE/ASRM-sponsored PCOS consensus workshop group. Revised 2003 consensus on diagnostic criteria and long-term health risk related to polycystic ovary syndrome (PCOS). Hum Reprod 2004; 19:41–7.

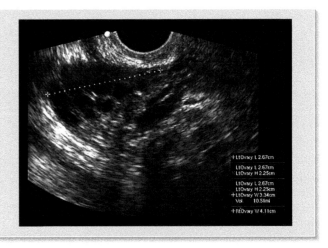

Amenorrhoea and oligomenorrhoea

Definitions: Amenorrhoea is the cessation or absence of menstrual periods and is defined as primary or secondary. Oligomenorrhoea is the term for infrequent menses. Bleeding occurs at intervals of more than 35 days (and less than 6 months). The causes, evaluation and treatment are similar.

- **Primary amenorrhoea:** failure to commence menstruation by 16 years of age with normal secondary sexual characteristics, or by 14 years of age in the absence of other evidence of puberty. The Tanner stages of pubertal development are used to assess development of secondary sexual characteristics
- **Secondary amenorrhoea:** absence of menstruation for ≥6 consecutive months in a woman with previously regular menses, or 12 months if she has previously had oligomenorrhoea
- The prevalence of amenorrhoea (not due to pregnancy, lactation or menopause) is approximately 3–4%
- Interruption of the hypothalamus-pituitary-ovarian (H-P-O) axis (see Fundamentals Figure 1.2) results in amenorrhoea
- Causes of primary and secondary amenorrhoea and oligomenorrhoea overlap (Tables 29.1 and 29.2)
- Secondary amenorrhoea is 40% ovarian, 35% hypothalamic and 5% uterine in origin. The commonest causes are PCOS, premature ovarian failure and hyperprolactinaemia

Complications

Women with amenorrhoea associated with estrogen deficiency are at increased risk of osteoporosis and may be at increased risk of cardiovascular disease. Infertility is a consequence of anovulation.

Management

- **History:** a thorough clinical history should include a menstrual history and drug history for medicines known to cause hyperprolactinaemia including recreational drugs (e.g. heroin). Enquiry about weight loss, stress and excessive exercise should be made. A history of uterine curettage should be noted, e.g. after miscarriage or abortion. Galactorrhoea may indicate hyperprolactinaemia which may be due to a prolactinoma
- **Examination:** BMI, signs of virilization, e.g. hirsuitism, male pattern baldness (may suggest an androgen secreting tumour); galactorrhoea; signs of thyroid disease
- **Investigations:** Pregnancy test, FSH/LH levels; prolactin; thyroid function tests (TSH); testosterone and free androgen index. Transvaginal ultrasound scan can identify polycystic ovaries, and confirm normal uterine anatomy
- **Referral** for further tests may be indicated based on the findings (Table 29.3). Karyotyping may be required for investigation of primary amenorrhoea and an abdominal rather than transvaginal ultrasound scan undertaken
- **Treatment** depends on the diagnosis and the individuals' concerns (e.g. infertility). Estrogen replacement is important to protect from osteoporosis. The COC can be used for this purpose assuming fertility is not required. Women with amenorrhoea and oligomenorrhoea occasionally ovulate spontaneously therefore contraception is recommended if pregnancy is to be avoided. Adolescent women with primary amenorrhoea may need artificial induction of puberty under the care of a specialized paediatric endocrinologist

Polycystic ovarian syndrome (PCOS) (Figure 29.1)

PCOS is a complex endocrine disorder and is the most common cause of secondary amenorrhoea. The cause is unknown and likely to be multifactorial. Hirsuitism, acne and obesity are common features and in many women insulin resistance and subsequent hyperinsulinaemia are key factors in the pathogenesis.

- **Complications:** impaired glucose tolerance and Type 2 diabetes; increased risk of cardiovascular disease, endometrial hyperplasia and endometrial cancer; infertility due to anovulation; association with sleep apnoea
- **Management:** this depends on symptoms. Lifestyle changes aimed at normalizing body weight can significantly improve symptoms. A weight loss of 5–10% can restore menstrual regularity. Menstrual cycle control is important to protect the endometrium and prevent hyperplasia. This can be achieved by using a COC in women who do not wish to conceive. The LNG-IUS is also a good option for endometrial protection. Acne and hirsuitism can be managed medically. Treatment of anovulatory infertility is usually by ovulation induction with clomifene citrate under the supervision of a fertility specialist. There may be a place for the use of insulin-sensitising drugs such as metformin however this is out with licence in the UK and should only be undertaken by a specialist

Dysmenorrhoea

- **Definition:** pelvic pain occurring at the time or shortly before menses. It is extremely common, affecting between 50–90% of menstruating women. Historically classified as primary (absence of identifiable underlying pathology), or secondary (associated with underlying pelvic pathology, e.g. endometriosis)
- **Aetiology:** primary dysmenorrhoea is thought to be due to the release of prostaglandins which increase contractility of the myometrium and cause cramping pain. Some women have gastrointestinal disturbance which is also thought to be a consequence of prostaglandin release

Management

- **History:** determine the onset of symptoms in relation to menarche and the presence of associated symptoms which may indicate underlying pathology, e.g. PCB, IMB, dyspareunia. Establish the impact on the woman's life
- **Examination:** perform an abdominal examination in all women. Pelvic examination is indicated unless the woman is an adolescent with a typical history of mild symptoms and has never been sexually active
- **Investigations:** STI screen if indicated. Pelvic ultrasound may be helpful particularly if a pelvic mass is suspected. It may reveal endometriomas, fibroids, hydrosalpinges or other abnormalities. Diagnostic laparoscopy may be required
- **Treatment:** if examination is normal then treatment can be initiated without further investigations (Box 29.1). Treat underlying pathology if present

Gynaecological problems in SRH

Figure 30.1 Symptoms of core PMD

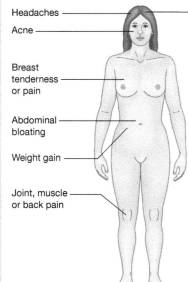

Headaches

Acne

Breast tenderness or pain

Abdominal bloating

Weight gain

Joint, muscle or back pain

Psychological
- Mood swings (e.g. feeling suddenly sad or crying, increased sensitivity to rejection)
- Irritability
- Depressed mood
- Anger, aggression
- Sleep disturbances
- Changes in appetite, overeating or specific food cravings
- Fatigue or lethargy
- Restlessness
- Poor concentration
- Social withdrawal
- Lack of interest in usual activities

Figure 30.2 Bartholin's abscess

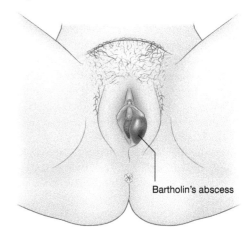

Bartholin's abscess

Table 30.1 Treatment of premenstrual disorders

Non-pharmaceutical treatments	Hormonal treatments (for ovarian suppression)	Non-hormonal treatments
Lifestyle modifications • Regular aerobic exercise, smoking cessation, alcohol restriction, stress reduction & dietary changes • Relaxation techniques • CBT	**Oral contraception** • Off-label if PMS is sole indication • Some evidence to support drospirenone-containing COCs, e.g. Yasmin	**Psychotropic drugs** • SSRIs, e.g. fluoxetine 20 mg daily continuously or luteal phase only • Or citalopram 10 – 30 mg/day
Supplements • Vitamin B6 • Vitex agnus-castus • Calcium carbonate • Magnesium oxide	**Gonodotrophin-releasing hormone agonist (GnRHa)** • Goserelin +/- add back therapy e.g. tibolone 2.5 mg/day	**Diuretics** • Spironolactone (100 mg/day during luteal phase)
	Gonadotrophin inhibitor • Danazol (200 - 400 mg/day)	**Anxiolytics** • Alprazolam • Buspirone
	Estradiol • Transdermal patches 100 – 200 mg/day (with endometrial protection e.g. LNG-IUS)	

Table 30.2 Treatment options for CPP

Analgesics
e.g. regular paracetamol, NSAIDs. Avoid opiates unless under the care of a pain management team

Adjuvant analgesia
Amitriptyline or Gabapentin may help neuropathic pain

Therapeutic trial of ovarian suppression
Useful for cyclical pain before offering diagnostic laparoscopy, e.g. COC, danazol, progestogens, GnRH analogues, LNG-IUS, for 3 – 6 months

Treatment for IBS
Antispasmodics, e.g. mebeverine hydrochloride and dietary modification if IBS suspected

Non-pharmacological therapies
e.g. TENS, acupuncture. No evidence of benefit although some women may find them helpful

Premenstrual syndrome (PMS)

Background

PMS is one of a complex group of conditions known as the premenstrual disorders (PMD). The International Society for Premenstrual Disorders (ISPMD) has redefined the classification of PMD, and PMS is now known as core premenstrual disorder.

Core PMD is a condition with distressing physical, behavioural and psychological symptoms regularly occurring in the luteal phase of the menstrual cycle and resolving during or shortly after menstruation to give at least one symptom free week. The severity of symptoms is great enough to cause significant impact on the quality of life.

- **Aetiology:** the exact cause is not known. The relationship with the luteal phase of the cycle suggests that the corpus luteum may produce a symptom-provoking factor
- **Symptoms:** over 200 premenstrual symptoms have been reported. Examples of typical symptoms are in Figure 30.1. Some women will suffer exacerbations of chronic illnesses, e.g. asthma, migraine, epilepsy
- **Diagnosis:** investigations are generally unhelpful. A detailed history including the timing of symptoms and any impact on the

Sexual and Reproductive Health at a Glance, First Edition. Catriona Melville. © 2015 by John Wiley & Sons, Ltd. Published 2015 by John Wiley & Sons, Ltd.
Companion website: www.ataglanceseries.com/sexualhealth

ability to function is important. The woman should be asked to keep a prospective symptom diary over at least two consecutive cycles. Several validated diaries exist, e.g. the Daily Record of Severity of Problems (DRSP). Patient-friendly internet-based systems are also available. For the diagnosis to be made, symptoms should disappear by the end of menstruation and recur in the luteal phase. They should also cause substantial impairment

- **Differential diagnosis:** depression, anxiety and panic disorders, hypothyroidism, irritable bowel syndrome and SLE are some conditions which should be excluded
- **Management (Table 30.1):** treatment should be tailored to the severity and type of symptoms and the woman's preferences. Progestogens or progesterone are not recommended. Surgery, i.e. bilateral oophorectomy and hysterectomy, can be considered under certain circumstances in secondary care

Dyspareunia

- **Definition:** pain during sexual intercourse. It can be classified as 'superficial' if pain occurs on penetration (often described as raw of burning) or 'deep' if pain is felt deeply in the pelvis occurring on deep penetration. Both types of pain can be present
- **Aetiology:** often multifactorial, for example vaginismus may develop as a consequence of discomfort due to a vulval dermatosis. Any pelvic pathology can present as deep dyspareunia, e.g. chronic PID, endometriosis
- **Assessment:** a concise history of the nature and onset of symptoms and any associated complaints, e.g. vaginal discharge or vulval itch
- **Examination:** look for signs of vulva changes, e.g. lichen sclerosus (LS), and any focal tenderness which might indicate vulvodynia. Tenderness over the uterosacral ligaments may suggest endometriosis
- **Investigations:** should be determined by the clinical findings. An STI screen, vulval swab for culture and sensitivity or pelvic ultrasound may be indicated
- **Management** depends on the underlying causes. Lubricants or vaginal moisturisers may be helpful, and referral for psychosexual therapy may be indicated. See sexual problems chapter for further information

Bartholin's cyst and abscess (Figure 30.2)

A Bartholin's cyst or abscess results from obstruction of the duct of the Bartholin's gland which provides vaginal lubrication. It affects about 2% of women in their lifetime. It presents as a unilateral cystic swelling in the posterior of the labium majus. Treatment is not usually required unless it becomes infected in which case an abscess can form which is tender, red and painful. The abscess develops in the lower third of the introitus but can expand anteriorly.

- **Management:** swabs from the abscess can identify *Neisseria gonorrhoeae* (in 20% of cases) and *Chlamydia trachomatis* so a full STI screen should be considered. Otherwise mixed vaginal flora are found
- **Treatment:** incision, drainage and marsupialization are undertaken. Antibiotics are not usually required unless there is surrounding cellulitis (or an STI is diagnosed). An alternative procedure is the insertion of a Word catheter under local anaesthetic

after incision of the abscess. It has an expanding balloon at the tip to keep the catheter in place

Acute pelvic pain

Can be due to gynaecological aetiologies, e.g. ectopic pregnancy, PID, ovarian cyst accident, or caused by gastrointestinal or urinary pathology. For assessment including investigations see Chapter 31, PID.

Chronic pelvic pain (CPP)

Chronic pelvic pain is an intermittent or constant pain in the lower abdomen or pelvis of at least 6 months in duration, not occurring exclusively with menstruation or intercourse and not associated with pregnancy. CPP is common, affecting one in six of the adult female population. CPP is a symptom, not a diagnosis and there are often multiple contributory factors.

- **Aetiology:** a wide variety of pathologies are associated with CPP e.g. endometriosis, adenomysis, adhesions from previous surgery or infection (PID), IBS and interstitial cystitis. Pain may be musculoskeletal in origin or due to nerve entrapment. Depression and sleep disorders are common in women with CPP and there may be complex psychological or social issues, e.g. a history of sexual abuse including domestic violence
- **Management:** a thorough history of the pain and associated symptoms should be taken. Explore the patient's fears and ideas about the source of the pain. Abdominal and pelvic examination may elicit tenderness, or reveal a pelvic mass (or may be normal). A pain diary can be helpful in recording symptoms
- **Investigations:** STI screen and/or urinalysis if indicated by the clinical findings. Likewise, pelvic ultrasound can be used to assess a suspected pelvic mass (however this may not be the cause of the pain). Diagnostic laparoscopy is now considered a second line investigation as it carries considerable risks and is negative in over one third of cases. Women may feel disappointed if no diagnosis is made following the procedure
- **Treatments:** underlying pathology should be treated. Other options are listed in Table 30.2

Additional resources

O'Brien PM, Bäckström T, Brown C, Dennerstein L, Endicott J, Epperson CN, et al. Towards a consensus on diagnostic criteria, measurement and trial design of the premenstrual disorders: the ISPMD Montreal consensus. *Arch Women's Ment Health* 2011;14:13-21

Royal College of Obstetricians and Gynaecologists. Premenstrual syndrome. Management. Green-top guideline 48. RCOG Press, 2007. www.rcog.org.uk/files/rcog-corp/uploaded-files/GT48ManagementPremensturalSyndrome.pdf.

Endicott J, Nee J, Harrison W. Daily Record of severity of problems (DRSP): reliability and validity. *Arch Women's Ment Health* 2006;9:41–9.

Royal College of Obstetricians and Gynaecologists (www.rcog.org.uk/files/rcog-corp/ManagingPremenstrualSyndromePMSInformationForYou.pdf)—Patient information leaflet on managing premenstrual syndrome

Royal College of Obstetricians and Gynaecologists. *The initial management of chronic pelvic pain*. Green-top Guideline 41. London: RCOG Press; 2012.

National Association for Premenstrual Syndrome (www.pms.org.uk)—Information and support for women with premenstrual syndrome

Pelvic Pain Support Network [www.pelvicpain.org.uk]

31 Pelvic inflammatory disease

Table 31.1 Factors associated with increased risk of PID

Risk factors for STIs	Age < 25 years Recent change of partner Multiple partners Lack of barrier contraception
Recent instrumentation of the genital tract	TOP IUD insertion within previous 6 weeks Fertility treatment Transcervical gynaecological procedures e.g. hysteroscopy, evacuation of the uterus
Past history of STI/PID/ ectopic pregnancy	

Table 31.2 Antibiotic regimens for PID

Outpatient regimen	Ceftriaxone 500 mg i.m. stat	*plus*	Doxycycline 100 mg b.d. plus Metronidazole 400 mg b.d. orally for 14 days
	or		
	*Ofloxacin 400 mg b.d. orally 14 days	*plus*	Metronidazole 400 mg b.d. orally for 14 days
Inpatient regimen	Ceftriaxone 1 g daily i.v. or cefoxitin 2 g i.v. t.i.d.	*plus*	Doxycycline 100 mg b.d. either i.v. (if available) or orally (if tolerated) plus Metronidazole 400 mg b.d. for 14 days
	Continue i.v. regimen until 24 hours after clinical improvement and then switch to: Oral doxycycline 100 mg b.d. plus metronidazole 400 mg b.d. for a total of 14 days		
Allergy	Azithromycin 1 g once a week orally stat for 2 weeks instead of doxycycline if allergy or tolerance are issues		

*Avoid ofloxacin if high risk of gonococcal PID (resistance).
Use doxycycline in place of ofloxacin if < 16 years old.
For current dosing regimens and recommendations consult BASHH guidance and BNF

Figure 31.1 Fitz–Hugh–Curtis syndrome

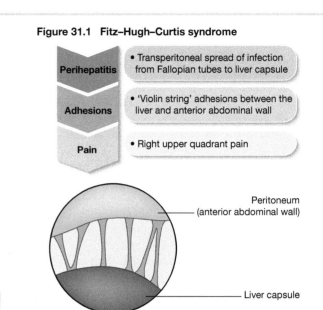

Perihepatitis	• Transperitoneal spread of infection from Fallopian tubes to liver capsule
Adhesions	• 'Violin string' adhesions between the liver and anterior abdominal wall
Pain	• Right upper quadrant pain

Peritoneum (anterior abdominal wall)

Liver capsule

Figure 31.2 Differential diagnosis of acute PID

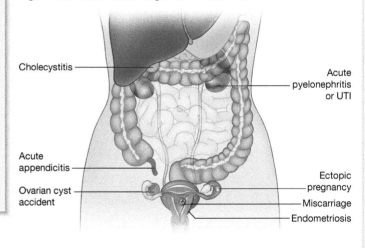

Cholecystitis

Acute pyelonephritis or UTI

Acute appendicitis

Ovarian cyst accident

Ectopic pregnancy

Miscarriage

Endometriosis

Background

Pelvic inflammatory disease (PID) is usually due to ascending infection from the lower genital tract. It can be either acute of chronic. It can cause endometritis, salpingitis, parametritis, oophoritis, tubo-ovarian abscess and pelvic peritonitis. The true prevalence is unknown but in the UK it is diagnosed in 1.7% of women aged 16–46 years annually, and in 15% of Swedish women in their lifetime. It is of clinical importance as it can have serious long-term sequelae.

- Aetiology: Causative agents include the STIs *Neisseria gonorrhoeae* and *Chlamydia trachomatis* which together account for a quarter of cases in the UK. Other microorganisms (all non-STIs) implicated are *Gardnerella vaginalis* and other anaerobes *(Prevotella, Atopobium and Leprotrichia)* that are commonly found in the vagina. *Mycoplasma genitalium* has also been associated with PID
- Genital tract tuberculosis is a rare cause
- Infrequently PID can be caused by direct spread of intra-abdominal infections, e.g. from appendicitis. Haematogenous spread has also been reported
- Associated risk factors are listed in Table 31.1

Clinical features

Symptoms
- Lower abdominal pain usually bilateral (can be subacute)
- Deep dyspareunia

Sexual and Reproductive Health at a Glance, First Edition. Catriona Melville. © 2015 by John Wiley & Sons, Ltd. Published 2015 by John Wiley & Sons, Ltd.
Companion website: www.ataglanceseries.com/sexualhealth

- Abnormal vaginal bleeding- including PCB, IMB and menorrhagia
- Abnormal vaginal discharge
- Backache
- Systemic illness with fever
- Nausea or vomiting (rare)
- Dysuria
- Can be asymptomatic

Signs
- Fever >38°C
- Lower abdominal tenderness (usually bilateral)
- Adnexal and/or cervical motion tenderness on bimanual examination
- Pelvic mass
- Purulent cervical discharge

Complications

A small delay in starting treatment causes a large increase in the risk of subfertility and ectopic pregnancy. Early antibiotic therapy reduces the risk of subfertility, ectopic pregnancy, and chronic pelvic pain

- Fitz–Hugh–Curtis syndrome occurs in 10–20% of women with PID (Figure 31.1)
- Infertility (tubal factor): repeated PID doubles the risk of tubal damage: one episode 8% risk; two episodes 19.5% risk, three+ episodes 40% risk
- Ectopic pregnancy: increased risk (sevenfold) correlates with severity and number of episodes of PID
- Chronic PID: irregular menses, dysmenorrhoea, deep dyspareunia, chronic pelvic pain, backache, malaise and fatigue

Diagnosis

The diagnosis of PID is made clinically. A low threshold for diagnosis and empirical treatment should be considered, especially for young sexually active women in view of the potential for serious morbidity. Other causes of pelvic pain should be considered (Figure 31.2).

- A positive result for chlamydia or gonorrhoea supports the diagnosis (but absence of these infections does not exclude PID)
- An elevated C-reactive protein (CRP) or ESR, pyrexia >38°C and leucocytosis may support the diagnosis
- Absence of cervical white cells on microscopy makes PID extremely unlikely (negative predictive value 95%) but their presence is non-specific

Investigations
- Pregnancy test: urine or serum β-hCG is essential for all women of reproductive age
- FBC, ESR/CRP
- Screening for STIs including HIV: NAAT for gonorrhoea and chlamydia; microscopy (if available); culture for gonorrhoea
- BP, heart rate and temperature if clinically unwell
- Transvaginal ultrasound scan may demonstrate free fluid, thickened dilated tubes or tubo-ovarian abscesses and can help exclude other causes such as ectopic pregnancy (EP)
- Laparoscopy is considered the gold standard diagnostic test but is an invasive investigation and not justified routinely

Management

General
- If severe disease, advise rest and consider admission to hospital for parenteral therapy
- Parenteral therapy is also advised if clinical signs of pelvic peritonitis or tubo-ovarian abscess
- Provide appropriate analgesia
- Advise no sexual intercourse until antibiotics completed and follow-up and PN undertaken
- Provide written information about the diagnosis and long term implications and explain that future use of barrier contraception will significantly reduce the risk of PID

Treatment
- Broad spectrum antibiotic therapy is required to cover *N. gonorrhoeae, C. trachomatis* and anaerobic infections (Table 31.2)
- Surgical management is occasionally indicated. Laparoscopy can be used for adhesiolysis or to drain pelvic abscesses, however ultrasound guided aspiration of pelvic fluid collections is a less invasive alternative. Division of perihepatic adhesions can be undertaken at laparoscopy but it is not known whether this improves the outcome when compared to antibiotic therapy alone
- *Special circumstances*
- **PID in pregnancy** is associated with an increased risk of fetal and maternal morbidity therefore parenteral therapy is advised. Tetracyclines should be avoided (use erythromycin instead) but otherwise the risks of the recommended antibiotic regimens are justified
- **HIV infected women** do not require a change to the standard treatment regimens as they respond well to these, even though they may have more severe symptoms of PID
- **Women with an IUD in situ**: The evidence as to whether an IUD should be removed in women with PID is limited and expert opinion is conflicting. Continuation of intrauterine contraception with current PID is awarded a UKMEC 2. Routine removal of the device is not recommended and removal should only be considered if symptoms fail to resolve within 72 hours of initiation of antibiotics, or if the woman requests removal. Hormonal emergency contraception may be required if removal of the device is planned

Partner notification
- Current sexual partners should be offered screening for gonorrhoea and chlamydia and epidemiological treatment with a broad-spectrum agent, e.g. azithromycin 1g stat oral dose
- The 'look-back' period for PID is 6 months but should be dictated by the sexual history

Follow-up
- Review moderate/severe disease at 72 hours to ensure clinical improvement. Mild cases should be reviewed at 2–4 weeks
- Follow-up should determine the resolution of symptoms and signs, compliance with antibiotic therapy and check PN
- The requirement for repeat chlamydia and gonorrhoea testing should be considered, e.g. non-compliance with antibiotics, persisting symptoms, possibility of reinfection

32 Menopause

Figure 32.1 Consequences of the menopause

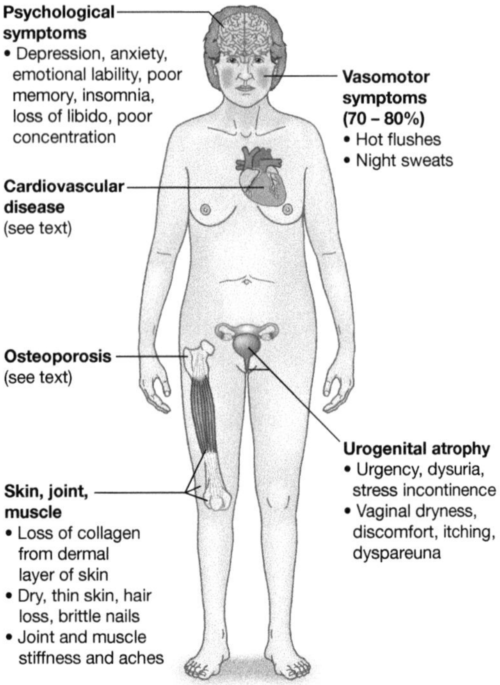

Psychological symptoms
• Depression, anxiety, emotional lability, poor memory, insomnia, loss of libido, poor concentration

Vasomotor symptoms (70 – 80%)
• Hot flushes
• Night sweats

Cardiovascular disease (see text)

Osteoporosis (see text)

Urogenital atrophy
• Urgency, dysuria, stress incontinence
• Vaginal dryness, discomfort, itching, dyspareuna

Skin, joint, muscle
• Loss of collagen from dermal layer of skin
• Dry, thin skin, hair loss, brittle nails
• Joint and muscle stiffness and aches

Table 32.1 Types of HRT

Treatments	Indications
Estrogen-only HRT	For women **without a uterus**, e.g. Elleste solo® 1 mg (oral), Estraderm MX® (patch), estradiol implant (rarely used due to tachyphylaxis and discontinued in the UK)
Sequential combined HRT	For women **with a uterus** and within 1 year of the LMP (or < 2 years after POF*). Progestogen is added for 12 – 14 days out of 28. One or 3-monthly regimens are available. A regular bleed occurs. e.g. Climagest® 1 mg
Continuous combined HRT	For women **with a uterus** who have been amenorrhoeic for > 1 year or on sequential combined therapy for > 1 year, or are aged > 54 years. 'Bleed-free' preparation. Any irregular bleeding should settle in 3 – 6 months (or will require investigation). e.g. Kliovance® (tablet), Evorel Conti® (patch)
Tibolone	A synthetic gonadomimetic with weak estrogenic, progestogenic and androgenic properties. In addition to treatment of vasomotor symptoms and prevention of osteoporosis, it may help libido. Does not stimulate the endometrium. 'Bleed-free' preparation
Androgen supplementation	Can improve loss of libido, particularly after surgically-induced menopause. There are few licensed options (implants and patches no longer available). Testosterone gel for male use can be used for female androgen replacement at a reduced dose (unlicensed)
Low-dose vaginal estrogen	For urogenital symptoms: tablet, pessary, cream, ring Vagifem tablet is licensed for long-term use; Estring® (ring) is licensed for 2 years. Each ring lasts 3 months
LNG-IUS	The Mirena® can be used as the progestogenic component of HRT for women with a uterus. Can be helpful for reducing side-effects associated with systemic progestogen and will provide contraception

Notes: HRT contains low doses of natural estrogens (as opposed to the high-dose synthetic estrogens in contraception). Micronized progesterone may be associated with a lower risk of breast cancer, cardiovascular disease and thromboembolic events than synthetic progestogens. Non-oral estrogen is associated with a lower risk of VTE and stroke. HRT does NOT provide contraception. *POF; premature ovarian failure.

Box 32.1 Contraindications to HRT

Unexplained vaginal bleeding

Pregnancy

Estrogen-sensitive cancer

Current, past or suspected breast cancer

Untreated endometrial hyperplasia

Active or recent arterial thromboembolic disease (e.g. angina or MI)

Previous or current venous thromboembolism

Untreated hypertension

Porphyria cutanea tarda

Active liver disease with abnormal LFTs

Box 32.2 Causes of premature ovarian failure (POF)

Unknown: there may be a family history

Chromosomal disorders: Turners syndrome, fragile X syndrome

Autoimmune disease: hypothyroidism, Addison's disease, diabetes mellitus

Infection: mumps, TB, CMV, malaria

Iatrogenic: radiotherapy, chemotherapy, surgery (oophorectomy)

Table 32.2 Alternative treatments to HRT

Treatments		Benefit
Lifestyle modifications	Exercise, sleeping in a cooler room, stress reduction, avoidance of spicy foods, caffeine, smoking and alcohol	May be suffcient to manage symptoms in some women
Non-pharmacological	Vaginal bioadhesive moisturisers, e.g. Replens®	Rehydrates the tissues and provides a reasonable alternative or adjunct to HRT
Pharmacological A-2 agonists	A-2 agonists e.g. clonidine can be used for vasomotor symptoms	Marginal effect over placebo for vasomotor symptoms
Antidepressants	Selective serotonin and noradrenaline reuptake inhibitors (SSRIs, SNRIs), e.g. fluoxetine® (SSRI), venlafaxine® (SNRI)	Beneficial effect for vasomotor symptoms
Anti-epileptics	Gabapentin®	Beneficial effect for vasomotor symptoms
Complementary therapies	Acupuncture, osteopathy, hypnotherapy, reflexology, Reiki, Tai Chi, mindfulness, CBT	Variable evidence of effectiveness. Further research is needed
Botanical therapies Plant estrogens	Phytoestrogens	Compounds found naturally in many plants, fruits and vegetables. Soy products and red clover may help vasomotor symptoms but long-term safety data is lacking
Herbal remedies	Dong quai, evening primrose oil, ginkgo biloba	Studies have not shown these therapies to be effective and there may be safety concerns and drug interactions
	Black cohosh	May help vasomotor symptoms but long-term safety data is lacking
	St John's wort	Effective in treating mild and moderate depression but many drug interactions

Sexual and Reproductive Health at a Glance, First Edition. Catriona Melville. © 2015 by John Wiley & Sons, Ltd. Published 2015 by John Wiley & Sons, Ltd.
Companion website: www.ataglanceseries.com/sexualhealth

Background

The menopause is the last spontaneous menstrual period and is due to the permanent cessation of ovarian function. The diagnosis is made in retrospect after 12 months of amenorrhoea. The fluctuations in hormonal levels associated with declining ovarian function usually begin in the fourth decade and last several years. This reproductive phase is called the climacteric, perimenopause or more recently the menopausal transition.

- The average age of the menopause is 52 years and by age 54 years, 80% of women will have stopped having menses
- Menstrual bleeding patterns change during the menopausal transition, with regular menses being replaced by erratic anovulatory cycles and episodes of amenorrhoea until the final menstrual period occurs

Consequences of the menopause (Figure 32.1)

- Physical, sexual and psychological symptoms are frequently reported in the early stages of menopausal transition
- Although psychological symptoms are reported by many women, there is a lack of evidence to support a causal relationship with the menopause. Depression and anxiety may be related more to psychosocial issues such as relationship or family problems, retirement or caring for elderly parents
- Mood changes can be secondary to sleep deprivation caused by night sweats
- The aging process itself may be responsible for some of the symptoms around the time of the menopause, e.g. decline in cognitive function

Symptoms:

- Occur due to the fluctuating and declining levels of hormones, and in particular the decreasing estrogen levels; 70–80% of women in the UK will experience menopausal symptoms
- Are usually self-limiting and resolve within 2–5 years, although vasomotor symptoms persist for many years after the menopause in 10% of women
- Can be debilitating in some women and severely impact on their quality of life
- Long-term consequences of the menopause are osteoporosis, urogenital atrophy and cardiovascular disease

Osteoporosis

- Estrogen plays a central role in maintaining the skeleton and there is a rapid decline in bone mineral density (BMD) following the menopause
- Almost 50% of women will have osteoporosis at 80 years of age and more than one in three women will sustain an osteoporotic fracture in their lifetime. The distal radius, neck of femur and thoracic spine (vertebral compression fracture) are the commonest sites of fragility fractures
- Osteoporosis is often asymptomatic and only diagnosed when a fracture occurs

Cardiovascular disease (CVD)

- Following the menopause, there is a marked increase in CVD. The exact mechanisms are still under debate as aging itself plays an influential role, however menopause is associated with an increase in body weight, redistribution of body fat and adverse changes to the lipid profile

Diagnosis of the menopause

- The diagnosis is made clinically. Investigations are rarely required and usually unhelpful. An exception would be FSH measurement in women using hormonal contraception (*see* Contraception for specific groups of individuals Figure 9.2)

Management of the menopause (Table 32.2, Box 32.1)

- Hormone replacement therapy (HRT) aims to replace estrogen after the menopause. Non-hysterectomized women require the addition of a progestogen to provide endometrial protection. Following a decade of uncertainty (primarily due to findings from the Women's Health Initiative (WHI) and Heart and Estrogen/Progestin Replacement Study (HERS)) regarding the safety and benefits of HRT, a global consensus statement was produced in 2013 which has provided clarity around the role of HRT
- For symptomatic menopausal women who are under 60 years of age or within 10 years of the menopause the benefits generally outweigh the risks
- HRT is the most effective treatment for vasomotor symptoms
- Urogenital symptoms: estrogen treatment is effective in treating vaginal and urinary symptoms related to atrophy. Low-dose vaginal preparations can be used long term with no requirement for added progestogen as there is no significant systemic absorption
- Osteoporosis: HRT prevents early postmenopausal bone loss and reduces fractures in postmenopausal women. The bone protective effect is estrogen dose related
- CVD: There appears to be a 'window of opportunity' whereby HRT commenced below the age of 60 years or within 10 years of the menopause reduces the incidence of coronary heart disease
- Stroke: the incidence of stroke (especially ischaemic strokes) is increased in some studies but the evidence is conflicting and the HERS study found no increased incidence of stroke with HRT
- VTE: oral HRT increases the risk of VTE 2- to 4-fold however the absolute risk is small and appears to be associated with oral rather than transdermal routes
- Breast cancer: The risk may be increased with use of combined HRT preparations for more than 5 years. The risk is related to many other factors including family history and BMI and decreases after treatment is stopped
- Ovarian cancer: risk is uncertain although there may be a small increase with use of HRT
- Cognition: evidence of the benefits of HRT is conflicting although some studies have shown an improvement in cognitive function with HRT started early in menopause

Routes

- Oral, transdermal (patch, nasal spray, gel, cream) topical/intravaginal, the intrauterine system; implants

Alternatives to HRT (Table 32.2)
Premature Ovarian Failure (POF) (Box 32.2)

- POF occurs in 1% of women under 40 years and 0.1% under 30 years of age. HRT is indicated until at least the average age of the natural menopause and is simply replacing the hormones which would have been produced at this age with no additional risks. HRT is necessary to control symptoms and reduce the risk of long-term health consequences e.g. osteoporosis

References and links

de Villiers TJ, Gas MLS, Haines CJ, et al. (eds) Global consensus statement on menopausal hormone therapy. *Climacteric* 2013;16:203–204.

de Villiers TJ, Pines A, Panay N, Gambacciani M. Updated 2013 International Menopause Society recommendations on menopausal hormone therapy and preventive strategies for midlife health. *Climacteric* 2013;16:316–337

www.thebms.org.uk the British Menopause Society

www.menopausematters.co.uk provides information about the menopause for patients and health professionals

www.daisynetwork.org.uk supports women suffering from POF

33 Sexual problems

Table 33.1 Causes of erectile dysfunction

Vasculogenic	Cardiovascular disease, HBP, hyperlipidaemia, diabetes mellitus, smoking
Hormonal	Hypogonadism, hypothyroidism, hyperthyroidism, hyperprolactinaemia, Cushing's disease
Neurogenic	Multiple sclerosis, Parkinson's disease, stroke, spinal disorders, surgery (of the pelvis), tumours, prolonged bicycling
Anatomical	Peyroni's disease, congenital curvature of the penis, hypospadias, epispadias, phimosis
Drugs	Antihypertensives, diuretics, antidepressants, antipsychotics, androgen inhibitors (treatment for benign prostatic hypertrophy), hormones, cytotoxics, recreational drugs, alcohol
Psychological factors	Depression, stress, relationship difficulties, previous sexual abuse

Box 33.1 Lifestyle modifications for ED

- Smoking cessation, reduction of alcohol consumption
- Weight loss including reduction of fat and cholesterol in diet
- Increased exercise
- Improved compliance with diabetes and cardiovascular medications
- Reduction of stress

Box 33.2 Treatment of vaginisimus

- Progressive relaxation
- Desensitisation (gradual introduction of vaginal trainers – Figure 33.1)
- Sensate focus
- Biofeedback with electromyography
- Hypnotherapy

Table 33.2 Treatments for erectile dysfunction

Serum testosterone	**Low (< 12 nmol/L)**	Testosterone replacement therapy
	Normal	**1st line** *Phosphodiesterase-5 (PDE5) inhibitors e.g. sildenafil (Viagra®), tadalfil (Cialis®), vardenafil (Levitra®) Vacuum erection devices
		2nd line Intracavernous injection therapy Intraurethral alprostadil
		3rd line Penile implant surgery (prosthesis)

*Sidenafil and vardenafil have a half-life of approximately 4 hours whereas tadalafil acts for up to 17.5 hours. A low dose should be prescribed initially with upwards titration as required. Before being classed as a non-responder to PDE-5 inhibitors a man should receive 8 doses at a maximum dose. These drugs are only available on an NHS prescription if certain criteria are met, e.g. multiple sclerosis, diabetes mellitus; otherwise a private prescription is issued.

Figure 33.1 Vaginal trainers

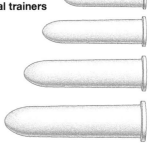

Table 33.3 Treatment for premature ejaculation

Pharmacotherapy	Short half-life SSRIs, e.g. dapoxetine 30 mg or 60 mg, taken 1 – 2 hours before sexual intercourse Conventional SSRIs, e.g. sertraline, fluoxetine, or TCAs e.g clomipramine (unlicensed) Tramadol (not recommended for routine use as potential for drug dependency) Local anaesthetics applied topically, e.g. lidocaine/prilocaine cream (unlicensed)
Behavioural therapy	Stop/start technique Squeeze technique Sensate focus
Psychosexual therapy	

SSRI = selective serotonin reuptake inhibitor
TCA = tricyclic antidepressant

Table 33.4 Physical causes of female sexual dysfunction

Disorders of female desire/arousal	
Depression	Drugs, especially antidepressants
Hormonal contraception	Vascular disease
Neurological disease	

Superficial dyspareunia
Infections, e.g. candidiasis, genital herpes simplex infection
Atrophic vaginitis
Genital dermatoses e.g. eczema, psoriasis, lichen sclerosus
Trauma, including post-natal
Other vulval conditions: vulval carcinoma, Behçet's disease

Deep dyspareunia	
Pelvic inflammatory disease	Pelvic adhesions
Ectopic pregnancy	Urinary or bowel conditions, e.g.
Endometriosis	irritable bowel syndrome, cystitis
Ovarian cyst	Pelvic malignancy

Table 33.5 Management of vulvodynia

General	Avoid aggravating factors and advise an emollient soap substitute
Topical local anaesthetic agents	e.g. lidocaine 5% ointment applied 15 minutes prior to and washed off just before sexual intercourse. Can cause local irritation so use with caution. May weaken latex condoms and if transferred to partner can cause penile numbness
Physical therapies	Addresses pelvic floor muscle dysfunction which is frequently present: • Pelvic floor muscle biofeedback • Vaginal transcutaneous electrical nerve stimulation (TENS) • Vaginal trainers
Pain modifiers	Amitriptyline, gabapentin, pregabalin, carbamazepine: benefit unclear, may be more helpful in unprovoked pain
Behavioural therapy	Cognitive behavioural therapy (CBT), psychotherapy
Acupuncture	Consider in unprovoked vulvodynia
Surgery	Modified vestibulectomy may benefit a minority of patients with provoked pain. Individuals who respond to lidocaine gel have better outcomes with surgery

Sexual and Reproductive Health at a Glance, First Edition. Catriona Melville. © 2015 by John Wiley & Sons, Ltd. Published 2015 by John Wiley & Sons, Ltd.
Companion website: www.ataglanceseries.com/sexualhealth

Background

Sexual dysfunction encompasses a variety of conditions affecting both men and women. It can arise from either physical or psychological causes or a combination of both. Problems with sexual function are extremely common as demonstrated in the third National Survey of Sexual Attitudes and Lifestyles (NATSAL-3), which found that >40% of men and >50% women reported sexual response problems in the preceding year.

Assessment

A thorough history should include the past medical and surgical history and drug history. The sexual history should include current and past relationship status and sexual orientation. Enquiry about smoking, alcohol, the use of illicit drugs and any stress at home or work should be made in the social history.

Sexual dysfunction in males

Erectile dysfunction (ED) (Tables 33.1 and 33.2 and Box 33.1) is the persistent inability to attain and/or maintain an erection sufficient for sexual performance. It is extremely common affecting ≥1 in 10 men in the UK. The prevalence increases greatly in older men. Risk factors for ED are similar to those for cardiovascular disease (CVD), including obesity, and a sedentary lifestyle. ED may be the first presentation of a serious underlying medical condition, e.g. HBP, as it may reflect a generalized arteriopathy associated with cardiovascular disease. Physical examination should include measurement of BP, heart rate, waist circumference and BMI. A genital examination is recommended. Investigations: all men should have serum lipids, fasting blood glucose, HbA1c and serum testosterone (measured on a blood sample taken between 8 a.m. and 11 a.m.). Prostate specific antigen (PSA) should be measured before starting, and during testosterone therapy. Referral for further assessment and management of CVD may be indicated. Management: identification and treatment of any curable causes of ED; lifestyle modification; psychosexual counselling. Men with a low total serum testosterone (<12 nmol/L) should have trial of testosterone replacement therapy. Surgery may be indicated for anatomical abnormalities.

Premature ejaculation (PE) is characterized by ejaculation which always or nearly always occurs prior to or within about 1 minute of vaginal penetration with the inability to delay this, (and has associated negative consequences, e.g. distress). The self-reported prevalence of PE may be as high as 25%. It is one of the most common male sexual problems and can occur at any age although shows a propensity for younger men. PE can either be acquired (secondary) or lifelong (primary). The aetiology can be divided into psychogenic causes, e.g. anxiety, relationship problems; and organic causes, e.g. chronic prostatitis, pelvic injury. Treatment includes pharmacotherapy, behavioural therapy and psychotherapy. A combination of these has been shown to be superior to individual treatments (Table 33.3)

Delayed or retarded ejaculation is the persistent or recurrent difficulty, delaying or absence of attaining orgasm (which causes personal distress). It can have a psychological cause or be due to an organic aetiology, e.g. spinal cord injury, diabetes mellitus or drug therapy. The mainstay of management is psychosexual therapy.

Sexual dysfunction in females (Tables 33.4, 33.5, Box 33.2)

Sexual problems in women are common. They can broadly be classified into disorders of sexual interest/arousal; orgasm; and disorders associated with pain. Sexual problems can be lifelong or acquired and generalized or only occurring in specific situations. Several problems can coexist; for example, dyspareunia can lead to arousal problems.

Disorders of sexual desire and arousal are commoner with aging and can be affected by hormonal influences e.g. the menopause. Psychosocial factors also play an important role including depression, stress and relationship problems. Failure to become physically aroused can be associated with peripheral neuropathy and spinal cord injury. *Anorgasmia* is more common in younger women. *Sexual pain disorders* include dyspareunia and vaginismus, which often occur together. Genital examination is necessary to exclude organic pathology, however several consultations may be required before the women is ready to be examined. Vaginisimus should be managed as a sexual pain syndrome.

Vaginismus is the persistent or recurrent difficulties of the woman to allow vaginal entry of a penis, a finger and/or any object, despite the woman's expressed wish to do so. There is often involuntary pelvic muscle contraction (of levator ani) and anticipation of pain. Factors such as negative beliefs about sexuality, or traumatising events, e.g. difficult childbirth have been implicated in the development of vaginisimus. Taking a concise sexual history and exploring the woman's thoughts about genital examinations can be helpful for diagnosis.

Vulvodynia has been defined as vulval discomfort, most often described as a burning pain occurring in the absence of relevant visible findings or a specific, clinically identifiable, neurological disorder. International Society of Vulval diseases (ISSVD) 2007

Classification: provoked, unprovoked or mixed. Generalized or localized.

Provoked vulvodynia: Unknown aetiology but probably multifactorial. There may be a trigger factor, e.g. a history of vulvovaginal candidiasis. Symptoms: vulval pain mainly at the introitus and felt at penetration, e.g. during SI or tampon insertion. Signs: no signs of acute inflammation; focal tenderness can be demonstrated by light touch with a cotton bud or swab. Diagnosis: clinical (also exclude other causes e.g. dermatoses). Investigations: STI screen if appropriate, ± skin swabs.

Complications: vaginismus, depression, relationship problems. Management: a combination of treatments can be helpful. If pain is provoked by sitting it may be due to pudendal neuralgia and referral to the pain team can be helpful. Remission can occur spontaneously in up to 50% of individuals within a year of diagnosis. Psychosexual referral may be required.

Unprovoked vulvodynia: Unknown aetiology. Symptoms: burning pain often longstanding and unexplained. It is commoner in postmenopausal women. Signs: normal vulva. Complications, diagnosis and investigations are as per provoked vulvodynia. Management: best managed as a chronic pain syndrome and pain modifiers in a titrating dose should be considered for initial treatment. Resistant unprovoked vulvodynia may need referral to a pain clinic.

Management of sexual dysfunction in females

Any underlying cause should be treated, e.g. estrogen for vaginal atrophy. Tibolone is licensed for treatment of loss of desire in postmenopausal women. Testosterone therapy can also be used in post-menopausal women who have no other identifiable cause of reduced sexual desire. Behavioural therapy and psychosexual therapy often have a role in management and some couples will require counselling for relationship difficulties.

Index

Note: Page numbers in **Bold** denote figures and tables